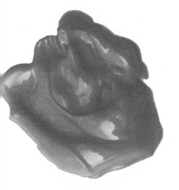

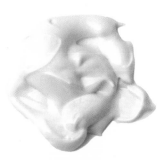

page 58

page 60

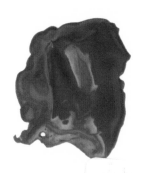

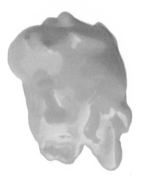

page

What's Your Baby's Poo Telling You?

What's Your Baby's Poo Telling You?

A Bottoms-Up Guide to Your Baby's Health

Josh Richman
and Anish Sheth, M.D.

AVERY
a member of Penguin Group (USA)   *New York*

Published by the Penguin Group
Penguin Group (USA) LLC
375 Hudson Street
New York, New York 10014

USA • Canada • UK • Ireland • Australia
New Zealand • India • South Africa • China

penguin.com
A Penguin Random House Company

Most Avery books are available at special quantity discounts for bulk purchase for sales
promotions, premiums, fund-raising, and educational needs. Special books or book excerpts
also can be created to fit specific needs. For details, write: Special.Markets@us.penguingroup
.com

Library of Congress Cataloging-in-Publication Data

Richman, Josh.
What's your baby's poo telling you? : a bottoms-up guide to your baby's health / Josh Richman
and Anish Sheth, M.D.
p.   cm.
ISBN 978-1-58333-543-7
1. Infants—Physiology—Popular works.   2. Infants—Health and hygiene—Popular works.
3. Feces—Popular works.   I. Sheth, Anish.   II. Title.

RJ125.R53   2014   2013050268
618.92'01—dc23

Printed in the United States of America
10   9   8   7   6   5   4   3   2   1

BOOK DESIGN BY NICOLE LAROCHE

This book is intended to help you better understand your baby (while also having fun). This
book is not designed to replace a real live pediatrician (we happen to know a few outstanding
ones, by the way). Please use this guide to help navigate your baby's barrage of bodily
emissions, but note that this book should not take the place of seeking medical treatment
when your child is sick.

To our parents for keeping our backsides clean.... It took us becoming parents to truly appreciate all you did for us.

~~~

To our friends and family for sharing their funny, scary, and peculiar experiences that inspired many of the entries in this book.

~~~

To our wives, Heather and Shilpa, two great moms . . . and one great pediatrician . . . for your encouragement and critical input for this book.

~~~

To our children, Samantha, Barrett, Rohan, and Ria, for providing endless inspiration (and material).

Contents

😵 **Doodie Disasters.** *These entries demand special attention, given their extreme nature. Survival is contingent on remaining calm, following instructions, and, whenever possible, calling your spouse for help.*

What's Your Baby's Poo Telling You?

Introduction

Newborn babies. They sure are cute, aren't they? Cuddly little dough balls that you just want to eat up. After all, what could be more precious than a mini version of you with pillowy soft skin and that hypnotic new-baby smell?

Before you get lost in the euphoria that is new parenthood, it is important to realize that raising a child is not one endless stretch of cooing and bonding. For the next few years, your waking life (what's left of it) will be consumed by dealing with your new baby's poo, pee, and gas.

At the risk of staining the porcelain-white image of babies everywhere, the time has come to break the seal of silence on baby poo. New parents may not be willing to look past a newborn's angelic attributes, while more seasoned parents will accurately depict these tots as potent excretion machines from the moment they are born. And most pediatricians will tell you that a baby's pee and poo provide critical indicators of a baby's overall health.

Sleep training? Vaccines? Forget it. The most important parenting decisions and signals involve poo. Will formula constipate my child? What is a normal number of bowel movements for a baby, anyway? Should I use cloth or disposable diapers? Is that red stuff in the diaper blood? How do I know when my child is ready to use the potty? The list of digestion-related queries goes on.

Adults who never cast a glance at their own waste will develop an intimacy with their own child's poo—looking, smelling, even touching their child's excrement to ensure its appropriateness.

While we do not recommend routine handling of poo, we applaud the efforts of parents everywhere to better understand their little bundles of joy by taking a look at what's in the nappy.

Congratulations, parents! This butt's for you.

One

A Survival Guide

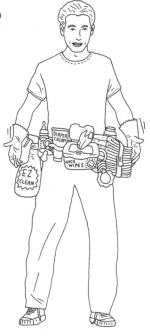

Some may cringe when we say raising a newborn is all about survival. Until now, life has been nothing but a field test. The SATs? College applications? Landing your first job? Navigating these life milestones will feel like mere practice missions.

It is now time for battle.

Don't let those chubby thighs and little fingers and toes throw you off your game. You are about to be bombarded with more poo, pee, gas, and vomit than you ever thought possible. Immediately after your baby is born, the first test will be deciphering poo's complex color code as you encounter jet-black, molasses-like stool unlike any you have seen before.

For most parents, the most daunting task will be dealing with the dreaded Poonami. This baby blowout will challenge even the most confident parents as they attempt to contain the incessant flow of diarrhea. Can you contain a Class III Poonami when faced with a wailing, thrashing child, in the shroud of darkness?

Your child will inevitably poo at the most inopportune time, in the most inconvenient place, and when you are least expecting it. How prepared are you?

Other bodily waste presents its own set of challenges. The art of burping encompasses not just getting your little one to bring up a little air after feeding but doing so in a way that prevents a spew of spittle from spoiling your entire wardrobe.

Combine this onslaught of bodily waste with an unimaginable dose of sleep deprivation you previously associated only with terrorist interrogations, and there should be no doubt that, yes, this is war.

This book will make sure you are ready to survive the barrage of excreta, regardless of the orifice of origin. We recommend paying special attention to those entries designated Doodie Disasters (indicated by the symbol ☻). Successfully navigating these high-stakes situations, often with the help of your spouse, will give you a sense of accomplishment while also minimizing dry-cleaning and carpet-cleaning bills.

Parents, prepare for battle. . . . There's no turning back now.

Two

Pregnancy and Poo

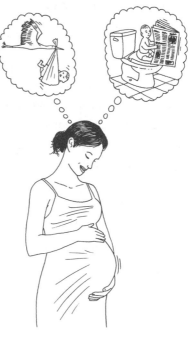

In the Oven

The miracle of life. We all marvel at those ten little fingers and ten little toes when we see them for the first time. And is there anything more special than hearing your baby's heartbeat or finding out if it's a girl or a boy (or twins!)?

Lost amid these admittedly poignant moments is the importance of the plumbing.

While the development of the digestive and urinary systems may not hold the cachet of the growing brain or heart, we would argue it is equally important.

Indeed, it is rare to hear new parents ask the ultrasound technician, "You know, seeing my child's beating heart was cool and all, but what we really want to see is our baby's rectum!" We would all rather think about those little fingers and toes or that cute little nose than consider the fact that our baby is swimming in *and* drinking her own pee. Yes, that's right. We call it *amniotic fluid* to make it sound sophisticated, but that fluid, which encapsulates our baby and comes pouring out of Mom during childbirth, is basically nine months' worth of recycled urine.

Poo, on the other hand, is a finely regulated waste product that accumulates inside the developing intestinal tract as the baby grows. This fecal material is composed primarily of dead cells and other debris and usually remains tightly sealed in the rectal vault until *after* birth (Meconium, page 45).

Despite the fact that pee and poo are ever present during fetal development, there is some comforting news regarding gaseous emissions; thankfully burps and farts only show up after birth.

Fetal Hiccups

Before feeling that first kick or first roll, most mothers-to-be will feel their baby hiccup in the womb. Also called *singultus*, fetal hiccups are a normal part of development caused by spasms of the diaphragm muscle, which helps control breathing. First felt in the early second trimester of pregnancy, hiccups can be one of the early bonding moments between mother and child. Hiccups can occur in infancy as well and are rarely a cause for concern, although some experts believe they occur when a young baby is overstimulated (loud noises, big crowds, etc.).

Pre-Baby Poo

A growing fetus inside a mother's womb brings many hopes, aspirations, and joys. It also wreaks havoc on the mother's digestive system. Pregnancy leads to a veritable poopourri of intestinal distress. Heck, even getting off the toilet seat can be a challenge in pregnancy's third trimester. Most first-time mothers-to-be are taken by surprise at these bodily malfunctions that begin at the time of conception and remain omnipresent until after delivery.

Your baby is something you are clearly looking forward to. Here are some aspects of pregnancy, however, that you could probably do without:

- Morning sickness, characterized by the not-so-joyful feelings and sounds of nausea, vomiting, and dry heaving
- Constipation—rock-hard, infrequent bowel movements

- Heartburn
- Frequent urination, i.e., needing to pee every ten minutes . . . with very little warning
- Engorged and inflamed hemorrhoids!

Most digestive problems can be blamed on two things. First, the increased pressure of a pregnant belly takes up space and displaces internal organs like the stomach and intestines, thereby affecting their function. Pressure on the stomach also leads to acid reflux as gastric juices back up into the esophagus.

The second factor, dare we say it, is hormones. High progesterone levels in pregnancy cause intestinal muscles to relax. These weakened muscles slow down digestion and the movement of stool, leading to constipation.

Most of these issues can be managed by eating smaller meals, drinking enough water, and, eventually, by delivering your baby.

Survival Tips (for Fathers-to-Be)

1. Read but do not repeat any of the Pregnancy and Poo chapter of this book. You can't understand what she is going through because you're not going through it.
2. Never use the words *disgusting* or *gross* in reference to your wife's pregnant body (or anything that comes out of it). You can't understand what she is going through because you're not going through it.
3. Even though this is one instance when you *can* blame your wife's hormones, don't do it. You can't understand what she is going through because you're not going through it.

The Mother Load

After sitting through high school health-class videos and, more recently, new-parent birthing classes, many expecant parents will feel well prepared for the excitement of the delivery room. One unexpected aspect of the birthing process curiously absent from all preparedness materials is the Mother Load, also known as the Special Delivery Poo.

The escape of stool from Mom is common during the pushing phase of delivery, especially if an epidural has numbed the entire pelvic area. With little sensation in the anal region, it can be impossible to sense an impending bowel movement (think about the uncontrollable drooling that occurs after getting numbed for dental work).

In addition to poo, several other not-so-savory items may come squirting out of women in the throes of labor. Frequent passage of flatulence and eruption of the amniotic fluid geyser are virtual delivery certainties, rendering the path to childbirth a messy one indeed.

First-time parents can be blindsided by these unpleasant aspects of delivery. Nurses and doctors, not so much. These trained professionals are clearly aware of the Mother Load. They arrive in the delivery room armed for combat, wearing protective gowns, face masks, even shoe covers. They have even been known to encourage mothers in labor by saying, "Push out your baby like you need to have a massive bowel movement!" (We are not sure this is the best way to motivate women to push forcibly, but, somehow, it works.)

Survival Tip (for Fathers-to-Be)

Stay at the head of the bed (if your wife will have you) and resist the urge to gaze downtown until the baby's head starts showing (we also would keep the video camera pointed elsewhere). Nothing good can come from peeking too soon. Most important, remain positive regardless of what kinds of bodily waste may escape. She *will* remember everything you did and didn't do during the agony of labor.

Remember, you're about to have a baby!

Postpartum Poo, aka the Afterbirth

Ahhh . . . a sigh of relief. You have just endured hours of hard labor, sweating, and grunting through the process of pushing out your newborn baby. It was tough, but well worth it! After delivering the baby, and then the placenta, you're still not done yet. There is one more delivery you will need to make. Let's hope this delivery will go smoothly (although it surely won't be as glorious, or as lovable).

The delivery in question is the Postpartum Poo. This first bowel movement after delivery can be just as painful (no epidural this time) and anxiety-provoking as having your baby. It can take a day or two, even longer, to successfully eliminate fecal matter after childbirth. Several factors conspire to make this a particularly dreadful experience. After hours of labor, women are dehydrated and fatigued. Surgical interventions such as a C-section or episiotomy can make going to the bathroom painful. Throw in some engorged, inflamed hemorrhoids from nine months of pregnancy and you have the perfect postpartum storm.

Survival Tip

All the above mentioned factors can conspire to cause a delay in having that first post-delivery bowel movement. When you're busy with more important issues like learning how to breastfeed and getting some much-needed sleep, the post-baby BM often takes, well, a backseat. Delaying the first bowel movement ends up making things worse; the longer stool sits inside the colon, the harder and more difficult it becomes to pass. Most physicians and midwives will recommend use of stool softeners and laxatives, if needed, in order to make sure new moms go early and often.

New moms: The passage of your Postpartum Poo signifies the return of normal intestinal function and *is* a reason to celebrate. We wouldn't go so far as naming or photographing this particular delivery, but there is nothing wrong with a quick high five for your nurse or husband (after hand-washing, of course).

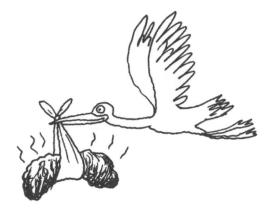

Three

Now That You've Had Your Baby, Here's the Essential Stool Box

The Wipe

Baby poo comes in many shapes and sizes. It may be rock hard or watery thin. Its aroma may be sweet or sour. After elimination, poo may come to rest in cloth or disposable diapers. Amid all this unpredictability remains one constant . . . the Wipe.

As wondrous as baby poo can be, it is, in the end, bodily waste that will be thrown in the trash. In developing countries, children are unhindered by diapers and are taught at an early age how and where to do the deed. In contrast, other cultures utilize diapers for the first several years of life to catch bodily waste. This practice allows us to move freely about our homes, unconcerned about stepping in would-be poo land mines.

Diapers, however, do have the downside of entrapping excrement against babies' butts, sometimes for hours at a time. Thus, adequate wiping of the backside, has become a necessary step in the diaper-changing process to ensure complete cleanliness.

Baby wiping is an essential skill that must be tailored not only to a baby's gender but also to the type of poo in question.

Here are some basic rules:

Wipe Type: Pretty basic, but important. While we all want our kids' butts to smell like a bed of roses, scented wipes can irritate the skin. The best wipes are alcohol- and fragrance-free.

Plan of Attack: Unless you are dealing with a Doodie Disaster (symbol 💀), most poo cleanups involve two geographic areas—the buttocks and the creases. Developing a proper plan of attack is crucial to success. Buttock cleaning should be done first before diving into the anal and thigh creases. Clean buttocks will allow you to relax your hogtie grip and lower your baby onto the changing pad without worrying about getting it dirty. If you are so inclined, once the butt cheeks have been cleaned, you can even lay down a fresh diaper while you tackle the crevices. If you have a chubby baby, make sure to scrape out poo remnants hidden amid those oh-so-cute thigh rolls. Overlooking these hidden areas can lead to infection.

The Backdrop

Even in the absence of a Poonami (page 78), a very common location for poo to settle is the lower back. Every diaper change requires an assessment of this easy-to-overlook area that is hidden from view while the baby is lying flat on her back. In order to see the lower back clearly you need to lift your kid by the ankles so she is practically standing on her head (she will

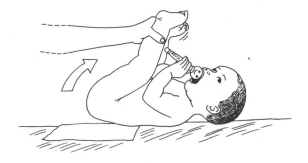

not like this). Alternatively, you can perform a blind sweep by reaching back under the buttocks and wiping in a downward motion. If it is clean, you are good to go. If poo appears, we recommend cleaning the buttocks first and then rolling your child on her side to finish the job.

Boys vs. Girls

We assume all new or expecting parents have an elementary-school-health-class level of knowledge regarding male and female anatomy. After all, you did figure out how to make a baby. A basic understanding regarding differences in male and female genitalia will also help you clean your child's poop without inflicting any collateral damage. Applied broadly, this means keeping stool off your furniture and your clothes. For your child, this means keeping fecal matter away from adjacent body parts.

Girls: Wipe front-to-back, making sure not to cross-contaminate genital areas with fecal residue. A good rule is to use a new wipe every time you come back to the front. Don't be cheap. Many parents will try to fold or crumple a used wipe to complete the job. Even if the wipe looks clean, just remember there are trillions of bacteria living in every gram of stool.

Boys: Wipe front-to-back or back-to-front. There is much less risk of genital contamination here. Why not go front-to-back for boys, also? Some feel the back-to-front motion offers increased shear force and, thus, better cleaning.

The Hyper-Wiper

Parents, especially new ones, can have trouble dealing with their newfound proximity to poo. The thought of seeing and smelling poo, let alone touching it, can drive parents to do outlandish things like wear rubber gloves or blow through half a packet of wipes during a single diaper change.

New parents can often be, well, anal when it comes to their child's cleanliness. The thought of a single streak or crumble being left behind is too much to bear. All of this can result in the practice of over-

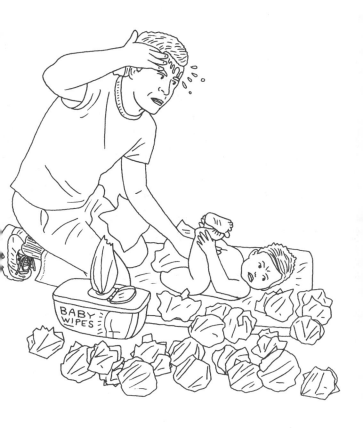

wiping. Remember, parents, you are cleaning your baby's skin, not scraping barnacles off the bottom of a boat.

The number of wipes needed per diaper change will decrease as you become more comfortable with poo's handling. By the second kid, you may grow comfortable using the diaper itself to hastily wipe the anal crease. Parents with three or more kids may become so at ease around poo that they will go half a day before noticing a poo remnant clinging to their shirtsleeve.

Bottom Line: A little poo left behind is no big deal. Don't obsess about removing every little poo particle from the anal crease. Overwiping can chafe a baby's skin and irritate the anal lining. Give the area a few gentle wipes, slap on a clean diaper, and live to fight another bowel movement.

No Wipes, No Problem

It's going to happen. You may be at home or at the park, but there will come a time when you need to change a dirty (and we are not talking about urine) diaper and have no wipes. The correct approach to this impending disaster is determined by when in the diaper-changing process you become aware of your lack of supplies.

If you realize you have no wipes prior to removing and discarding the old diaper, you are in luck. Keep Junior in his dirty diaper a little longer while you craft wipes by gently wetting a paper napkin or toilet paper with water, or with spit if that's the only option. (Tissues are a last resort as they tend to fall apart when wet.)

If you are already in the midst of the diaper change when you realize you don't have any wipes, things get a little more interesting. Given the laws that govern being a new parent, you will most certainly be alone when this happens. Also, it's a good bet that your child will be crying uncontrollably and that you are down to your last clean diaper. So what do you do?

Survival Tip

If you're changing a dirty diaper outdoors without wipes, resist the urge to use leaves, grass, or tree bark. Not only is this unsanitary, but the chafing that will result from using these rough "wipes" will not be appreciated by your little one. You may be able to use the *outside* of the dirty diaper to wipe the buttocks, but you will still need something for the crease. In this situation, something will have to be sacrificed. The best option is to sacrifice your baby's onesie or one of your own socks and go to town.

Worst-case scenario? Use water and your hand to clean it the old-fashioned way.

The Diaper

Former ESPN anchor Dan Patrick made famous the saying "You can't stop him, you can only hope to contain him." Most commonly used in reference to a star athlete playing at the top of his game, this aphorism, it turns out, applies equally well to the world of baby poo.

Baby poo is destined to come and come often. Your job over the next few years will be to limit its effect on your life. This all starts with the diaper.

Poo Goes Green? Cloth vs. Disposable Diapers

Most parents will toy with the idea of "going green" and using cloth diapers before their baby is born. Soon thereafter they are faced with the cruel reality of needing to wash up to a dozen diapers a day. Needless to say, most parents choose disposable diapers.

Turns out going cloth may not be all that better for the environment if you take into account the detergent, water, and energy usage needed for cleaning. Hybrid diapers involve disposable, flushable liners with cloth on the outside. But frankly, who has the time to take apart a dirty diaper?

In favor of disposable diapers are their enhanced absorptive capacity compared to cloth (thanks to the sodium polyacrylate crystals found in the diaper lining). This may help prevent diaper rashes by keeping your baby's butt drier for longer.

So is there any downside to disposable diapers aside from their impact on landfills? Because they are more absorbent and comfortable than cloth diapers, toddlers in disposable diapers tend to be potty trained later than their cloth diaper–wearing counterparts.

At some point, the choice between cloth and disposable diapers may become a lot easier for the busy, environmentally conscious parent. There are new efforts to commercialize compostable diapers, providing the ease of disposable diapers without contributing to landfill waste. We can't attest to their absorbency or comfort levels, but if done right, they could represent the next innovative step in advancing diaper technology.

The Application: Tight vs. Loose

Diaper snugness is a common cause for debate among new parents. Some parents will strap on a diaper as if they were cinching a corset, while others will leave it hanging loosely across the back and thighs.

The correct approach is dictated by your baby's set of circumstances. If diarrhea is flowing fast and furious, you may want to strap the diaper on tightly so as to try to prevent leakage around the thigh holes or up the back (Poonami, page 78). Conversely, if your child has a diaper rash, you may want to minimize skin moisture and allow air to dry the backside. This calls for a more loosely applied diaper.

Survival Tip

In general, diapers should be snug when applied, understanding that they will sag a bit as they get heavier with pee and poo. If your baby is having really bad diarrhea, you may want to consider the double-diaper dike technique and layer one diaper inside another to create an extra line of defense against leakage.

While it should go without saying, the top of your baby's butt crack should never be visible at the time of diaper application. As cute as this may seem, a visible butt crack is asking for trouble.

Diaper Disposal

Clean buttocks and a happy baby are good things. But the job does not end there. Regardless of your choice of diaper disposal contraption, you (or if you're lucky, your spouse) will ultimately have to discard a trash bag full of dirty diapers. As the diapers pile up and the pail approaches maximum capacity, each additional diaper becomes increasingly difficult to throw away.

It is commonplace for parents to resort to various techniques, including shaking and tilting the diaper receptacle, sometimes even resorting to brute force, in order to delay the inevitable fate of having to take the bloated bag of smelly diapers outside.

The time will come, however, when it becomes physically impossible to squeeze in even one last diaper. When that time comes, successful disposal of the trash bag full of diapers is critical; doing this improperly can spread horrific odors, which will linger throughout your house.

Survival Tip

Take the diaper pail out of the room, preferably out of the house, before opening it up to remove the trash bag. *Under no circumstances should you squeeze the air out of the bag before tying it off!* Doing so will result in a pressurized expulsion of lethal vapors directly into your face, not to mention your psyche.

After the bag is tied up and properly disposed of in the outside trash bin, consider spraying air freshener into your diaper receptacle before you bring it back inside. Extremely poo-smell-a-phobic? Consider placing a stick-on air freshener on the inside of your diaper receptacle to wage constant combat against that dirty diaper smell.

Some parents have gone so far as instituting a "no poopy diaper in the diaper contraption" rule, where only wet diapers are allowed to be disposed of indoors. This excessive rule mandates that all solid-waste diapers be immediately taken outside.

All Hands on the Poop Deck

Early-life diaper changes are easier from one perspective: Newborn babies don't move all that much. As the months go by, however, their mobility increases. By age three to four months, some babies will start to roll over, and soon after that they will learn to crawl and eventually stand up and walk. We celebrate these movement milestones and commemorate them in baby books and with posts to our Facebook pages.

This newfound mobility also has implications for safety. Electrical outlets should be plugged, baby gates should be installed at the top of stairs, and sharp table corners should be padded. Vigilance during diaper changes is also crucial. Leaving your newly active child unattended on an elevated changing table can be dangerous. The older your child gets, the less time she will need to unexpectedly wriggle free and roll off the changing table.

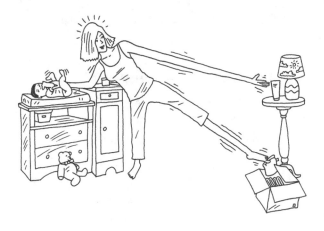

Survival Tip

Maintain hand control at all times. Be sure to keep at least one hand on your child while she's on the changing table. It's also a good idea to make sure you have all you need—wipes, diapers, etc.—within reach before beginning.

If for any reason you need to leave the changing area mid-diaper change, do not leave your baby alone on the table. Take her with you. Even if she is without a diaper, it is better to risk getting peed on than risk baby head trauma.

If your kid is *really* active during diaper changes, you may want to abandon the changing table altogether and change her diaper on the floor, pinning her legs down with your own.

Don't Wear White after Labor Day

Babies poop. Often at the most inopportune times.

Too often, just as you're ready to leave for work, you get a whiff signaling that your baby has just taken care of business. You briefly consider taking him to day care in his poopy diaper before parental guilt sets in. You check your watch and confidently proclaim, "I'll quickly take care of this," as you carry your sweet offspring to the changing table.

Pre-work diaper changes are fraught with collateral damage. The combination of a cleanly pressed long-sleeved shirt and dangling tie with a hasty diaper change frequently results in poo ending up where it shouldn't be.

Pressed for time, most parents will hurriedly tear off the old diaper and strap on a new one. Heading off to work with a sense of accomplishment, they fail to notice the presence of unexpected residue on their clothing.

Poo stains on the shirt cuff or lapel are typical battle scars resulting from morning encounters with dirty diapers. In the morning rush to get out the door, this collateral damage often goes unnoticed until later in the day, when a colleague points out the presumed "coffee" stain on your clothing.

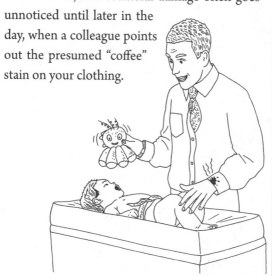

Survival Tips

1. Roll up your sleeves before beginning the diaper change. This simple step will ensure you don't end up with a poo-spotted sleeve.
2. Dads, take off or tuck in your tie. Not even the most dexterous daddy diaper changer can prevent tie contamination when it is loosely dangling over a baby's bum.
3. If needed, don an apron or smock to cover up work clothes.
4. This is no time to be a tree hugger. Use an ample wad of wipes to ensure that your wrists, as well as watches and bracelets, do not come in contact with poo.
5. Regardless of your protective techniques, be sure to perform a thorough self-inspection before heading off to work.
6. If colleagues notice the presence of poo on your attire while at work, blame it on spilled coffee.

Four

The Hue
of Poo

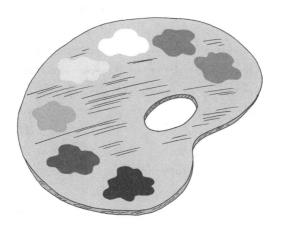

Poo Palette

Doo-Doosclaimer

Much of parenting anxiety these days stems from concerns about whether our child is "normal." Some may incorrectly assume that a child who enjoys smearing her feces on the wall is destined to become a social deviant. This can be totally normal behavior (and you can breathe easier knowing that her choice of finger paint is organic and lead-free) (Poocasso, page 122).

Just as with baby behavior, baby poo's range of normalcy is also quite broad. If there is one rule of baby poo, it is that no two days are alike. One day can bring seven bowel movements, the next none. Even going several days without a BM can be normal. Keep in mind that what is normal for your friend's child may not be normal for yours.

The Poo Palette is meant to entertain while educating. Baby poo can be pretty much any color and will change early and often. Pay attention to poo, but view your baby's poo in the context of how she looks. If she is eating and smiling and growing, chances are there is nothing to worry about.

It is commonplace for parents to rush their child to the ER or pediatrician's office concerned about their babies' bloody stools, only to find out the crimson color is the result of a healthy helping of beets (or Kool-Aid!).

Bottom Line: Most variations in poo color are benign, and remember, what goes in must come out!

Poovolution

Poo's dramatic color changes in life's first few days would make Jackson Pollock jealous. Keeping track of what's normal and what's not is one of the earliest (and most daunting) tasks of parenthood.

Just when you start getting used to seeing that dark, sticky stool known as meconium (which you can now proudly pronounce correctly), you are faced with a barrage of colors and consistencies that leave you wishing all poo was soft, formed, and brown.

Throw into this poopourri things termed *seeds* and *curds*, and one begins to wonder how such a small, seemingly innocuous, little human being can produce such a mind-boggling array of waste. *And* this all takes place before your little one starts eating regular food!

As a general rule, poo does tend to lighten up in color and consistency over the first week or so of life, evolving from black and tarry to green to yellow before finally settling down to the familiar brown hue we have come to know and, um, love.

Black
Meconium
This tarry, black, remarkably odorless product is usually expelled in life's initial twenty-four hours. Meconium shares its color and consistency with Marmite, the yeasty British spread, but thankfully lacks its pungent aroma (we aren't sure about the taste).

Meconium passage is an important milestone unto itself. Adult poo resides in our intestinal tract for only a few days, whereas meconium has been in a newborn's digestive pipeline for nine months (well, almost). Meconium is made up of dead intestinal cells, swallowed amniotic fluid debris, bile, and various gastrointestinal enzymes and basically represents the sum total of digestive waste from a baby's time in the womb.

If meconium is prematurely passed into the amniotic fluid while the baby is still in the womb, it can be dangerous. Premature meconium passage occurs when there is fetal distress during childbirth, or more frequently in overdue babies (delivered after the forty-second-week mark), and is often first discovered when a mom's "water breaks" and the fluid is found to be darker than normal.

Inhalation of poo particles into the newborn's lungs can lead to a breathing problem known as meconium aspiration. Prompt suctioning of meconium from a baby's airways is needed to prevent serious lung problems.

In most healthy newborns, meconium is passed

within twenty-four hours of the first feeding. When this lustrous, ebony-hued poo comes, make sure you have enough wipes on hand. Meconium's sticky, glue-like consistency coupled with a new parent's fixation on having a baby with a sparkly-clean butt can equal the need for a dozen or more wipes at a time.

Be aware that delayed meconium passage can be the first sign that something is wrong with a baby's digestive system. The lack of a dirty diaper in the first few days after birth may seem like a blessing amid the sleepless nights and other hardships of early parent-hood, but it can sometimes be a sign that your baby's plumbing is not working properly. Should you cher-ish the lack of diaper changes or call for help? It is probably a good idea to alert your pediatrician if your baby doesn't poo in the first twenty-four to forty-eight hours.

A much less common cause of jet-black stool is in-ternal bleeding from the stomach. Blood, when orig-inating from high up in the intestinal tract (i.e., the stomach), turns black and tarry and is called *melena*.

This sort of bleeding is rare in newborns but should be kept in mind if black stools show up after the first few days of life.

Note to parents: Inhale deeply while changing meconium-filled diapers and savor the (lack of) aroma. Failure to do so will lead to deep regret when you realize that all future diaper changes involve poo with smells ranging from putrid to abhorrent. (Note: Breast-feeding can keep baby poo's stench temporarily under wraps; see below.)

Yellow
Breast-Fed Poo

Among the many reasons to choose breast milk over formula-feeding is the sweet-smelling poo it produces. Many have likened the smell to buttered popcorn. Okay, so breast milk poo's aroma may not exactly rival that of the corner bakery, but it is infinitely more tolerable than formula poo's stale-milk stench. The yellow, seedy appearance of breast-fed poo brings to mind a certain Rolls-Royce–commercial-made-famous Dijon mustard. (*Pardon me, would you happen to be breast-feeding your child?*)

The gastrointestinal tract of a breast-fed infant is a well-oiled machine. Poo comes fast and furious, often up to six times a day. In contrast, formula-fed babies put out three or four (much smellier) bowel movements a day.

Breast milk's carbohydrates and proteins are easily digested by a baby's developing small intestine, leaving less residual matter for processing in the colon when compared to formula. This results in a less bulky, more watery, and more frequent stool. Its easy processing also explains why breast milk poo doesn't smell all that bad (there is less debris in the large intestine for bacteria to ferment).

Breast milk comes in a few different varieties, each vintage providing your baby with much-needed nutrients.

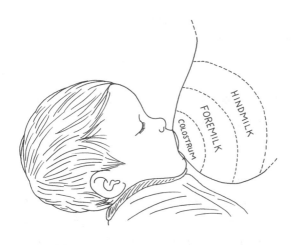

Colostrum

Also known as "liquid gold," this early breast milk vintage is produced in the days leading up to delivery and dries up in about seventy-two hours. Small in quantity but high in protein, this "power shot" is not unlike the energy gels used by long-distance runners. Colostrum is concentrated goodness, full of nutrients crucial for the gastrointestinal (GI) tract and immune system.

Mature breast milk takes several days to a week to come in and is composed of foremilk and hindmilk.

Foremilk

A refreshing thirst quencher, foremilk is higher in water content and lower in fat. This milk is usually delivered in the first few minutes of feeding and will satisfy your baby's thirst.

Hindmilk

A rich, creamy milk that delivers high-caloric content and creates satiety. Hindmilk begins flowing after foremilk has dried up and makes up the last two-thirds of the feeding. It is best thought of as a "power smoothie," filling up your baby's tummy and creating that blissful post-meal state known as a food coma.

Breast Milk versus Formula Composition

	Breast Milk	**Formula**
Protein	7 percent	15 percent
Fat	55 percent	50 percent
Carbohydrates	38 percent	35 percent
Smell when deposited in diaper	Buttered popcorn	Stale milk

Doo You Know?

- An infant can effectively drain all the breast milk from a single breast in seven minutes!
- Newborns can be lazy! In fact, the "lazy baby syndrome" refers to babies who basically lie around and do nothing for the first twenty-four hours. Mothers often grow concerned that the lack of feeding means their babies are not getting enough nutrition. The truth is that babies don't need much more than a shot of colostrum every now and then in the first day of life. Their vigor and appetite usually pick up by

day two or three. The bad news? You'll have to wait a few more years for them to start helping around the house.

- Nature's elegance: A human baby doubles its weight by four months of age. This is three times longer than a calf's growth rate (calves double their weight in less than two months!). To allow for this more rapid growth, Mother Nature has customized cow's milk to contain three times more protein than human milk (3.5 grams/dL vs. 1.1 grams/dL).

Green
Guacapoo

There's nothing like a healthy helping of extra chunky guacamole to go with that spicy beef and cheese burrito. Finding a green semisolid load that looks like your favorite Mexican side dish in your baby's diaper, however, is an altogether different scenario. Instead of reaching for the nearest tortilla chip, you will be looking for an ample supply of baby wipes and the nearest changing table.

Like most shades of baby poo, green stool can be normal. Dark green stool is typical after giving your baby iron-fortified formula or other supplements containing iron. In addition, breast-fed babies can churn out green stool if they are "snacking" on watery foremilk. A diet made of mostly foremilk leads to green stools and an unsatisfied baby. Switching kids from one breast to the other too quickly during breast-feeding can deprive them of rich, fatty hindmilk. Hindmilk is like a milkshake that will leave your baby feeling content and change green stools into yellow, seedy bowel movements.

Viral and bacterial infections of the GI tract are more concerning causes of seaweed-looking green stool. Green infectious diarrhea can be severe with liquid poo being discharged at a rapid rate, leaving little time for dallying during diaper changes. When this green goblin rears its ugly head, minimize your baby's air time. *Green means Go*. Slap down a clean diaper as soon as you peel off the old one. Failure to do so can lead to disaster. And trust us, it's no fun trying to explain to your spouse how this seaweed soup ended up on the new Persian.

Bottom Line: If your baby's poo is green but not particularly loose, try increasing the time she spends feeding at one breast before switching her over to the other. To ensure your child finishes off all the hindmilk in each breast, start each feeding on the breast your baby last fed off. This will ensure that any hindmilk left behind from the previous feeding is fully drained. An ample intake of hindmilk will turn poo back to its customary yellow color.

If stool is flowing fast and furious and resembles green seaweed, there's a good chance your baby has a gastrointestinal infection. Keep your child hydrated, change diapers quickly, and consult your pediatrician.

Brown

The color brown has become synonymous with adult poo. Adult stool's brown color comes from the presence of stercobilinogen, a compound created when intestinal bacteria digest bile. Pediatric poo can be brown early in life but is largely overshadowed by black and then yellow stools, especially in breast-fed babies. Most any shade of brown can be seen in the evolution of healthy baby poo, tan being the most common. Formula-fed babies tend to transition to tan/brown stools more quickly when compared to their breast-fed counterparts, who remain in the yellow end of the color spectrum until they begin to consume solid foods.

Kids grow up fast. So savor the days of colorful poop. Seeing brown consistently in your kid's diaper means his digestive tract is starting to work like yours. It will seem like in the blink of an eye he will be asking to borrow your car keys!

Maroon

Currant Jelly

In keeping with the likeness between poo and things you spread on toast (e.g., Marmite, Dijon mustard), the appearance of this thick, dark red stool is classically described as "currant jelly." For those less sophisticated readers, currant is a type of berry. Currant jelly is made by boiling currants with sugar until you have a gelatinous mixture akin to raspberry jam. It sure sounds yummy. . . .

Currant jelly *stool*, on the other hand, is not quite as flavorful. It is a mixture of fecal material, blood, and mucus and is seen in kids who have a particular kind of bowel blockage called intussusception. This condition can occur beginning around six months of age and becomes less common after age three. Intussusception is caused by one intestinal segment telescoping into another, causing a blockage that results in abdominal distention, fussiness, and vomiting.

Bottom Line: If your baby's poo is maroon and resembles currant jelly, you should go to your pediatrician for further examination. Diagnosis of intussusception is made by a barium X-ray, and surgical treatment is sometimes required.

Rotavirus is one of the most common causes of vomiting and diarrhea in young children. The hallmark of this viral infection is massive amounts of diarrhea (sometimes upward of fifteen to twenty bowel movements a day!). Not only does this illness do a number on the diaper budget, it can cause serious dehydration and even hospitalization. This infection also happens to be the number one cause of the feared Poonami (page 78).

Sounds like something worth preventing, doesn't it? Turns out the original vaccine was very effective in preventing rotavirus infection but also caused higher rates of intussusception (and currant jelly stool) and was pulled from the market. Thankfully, there are now two second-generation vaccines that do not appear to have the same side effects. Rotavirus vaccines are, once again, recommended for all infants.

White

This poo can be difficult to see as it blends in with a diaper's white background. While you may be eager to reseal the diaper and declare a false alarm, closer inspection will reveal pale-colored stool not unlike a dollop of soft-serve vanilla ice cream.

Poo can be many colors, but it should never be white. Short-lived pale white stool is most often due to a viral infection. This color change will typically last a day or two, at most.

White poo that is persistent can be a sign that bile excretion from the liver is being blocked. Bile is poo's natural food coloring; it is what gives poo its green and brown coloration. If the pipes that pump bile into the intestines become blocked, the end result is color-less poo (think of a snow cone without any flavored syrup).

Bottom Line: Persistent, pale white stools should prompt a visit to your pediatrician. Blood work and imaging tests (i.e., CT scan, ultrasound) will reveal the underlying cause and lead to treatment that will restore bile's normal flow.

All white stuff that ends up in the diaper is not poo.

Leave it to Mother Nature to throw you a curveball (just when you were starting to feel comfortable with poo's multitude of colors and consistencies).

Babies emerge from the womb looking like they are smeared in condiments. Amid the blood and mucus is a substance called vernix, a white, greasy paste not unlike cotija cheese. This slimy layer of gunk helps protect a baby's skin while it swims in the womb for nine months.

Vernix is quickly washed off during the baby's first bath, but remnants can linger in the genital region (especially in girls) for a few days after birth. Frequently encountered stuck in thigh folds and butt creases, vernix is not harmful to the baby and will likely disappear completely after a thorough cleaning. Some have even advocated delaying a newborn's first bath to allow this cheesy body scrub more time to prepare the skin for life outside the womb.

Baby Blue

The rarest and most shocking hue of poo has to be blue. When it comes to the human body, the color blue is rarely seen anywhere outside the eyeball and, occasionally, on the skin. So when it shows up in your baby's diaper, you know it must be coming from something your child ate. The most common culprit, not surprisingly, is, yes, *blue*berries. Beyond this, artificially colored items such as juices and Popsicles are usually to blame.

Bottom Line: Baby-blue poo is always diet-related. If your kid inhaled a Cookie Monster cupcake at a birthday party, expect blue poo a day or two later.

Red

Red is a color that belongs on roses, Twizzlers, and Christmas sweaters. It doesn't belong in your newborn baby's diaper. Or does it? Red, more than any other poo hue, can strike fear in the hearts of new parents.

Thankfully, traces of blood seen in the infant diaper are mostly due to benign conditions. Among the most common reasons for bleeding is an anal fissure, a small cut in the sphincter muscle that develops after passage of a particularly hard bowel movement. Children may appear to be in pain while straining or may avoid having a bowel movement altogether. The mainstay of treatment to keep stools soft is having a baby drink small amounts of diluted prune or pear juice. Petroleum jelly can be applied to the tear to help ease the discomfort.

Milk protein allergy is a unique cause of red poo seen in infants who are intolerant of certain proteins found in cows' milk (Dairy Doo, page 114). Inflammation in the intestines causes bleeding, and treatment consists of eliminating cow's milk from the baby's and mother's diet if she is breast-feeding.

As with all poo color changes, one must examine the child's diet for the preceding twenty-four hours. Did Junior scarf down a cherry Popsicle? Froot Loops? Beets? Quite often, short-lived red stool can be traced back to consuming red food.

Other times, red debris in the diaper may have *nothing* to do with poo at all.

Baby Vampire

Believe it or not, childbirth can be a traumatic process and babies can actually swallow Mom's blood during delivery. Swallowed blood will usually appear a darker shade of red (or black) by the time it makes its way into the diaper.

Babies can also swallow Mom's blood during breast-feeding when dried, cracked nipples are present. Bleeding from small cracks in Mom's nipples is subtle and may occur only while the baby is nursing. In cases where the bleeding source is unclear, medical tests can determine whether the blood is coming from the mom or baby.

Pink Pee

In the era of superabsorbent diapers, it is rare to see any liquid in the nappy. We can tell our child has peed by the change in diaper weight and, of course, by recognizing the characteristic diaper sag. In some instances, however, urine does leave its mark. Uric acid crystals stain the diaper pink and are seen in the first few days of life when breast milk production is low. These pink crystals signify dehydration and will disappear from your baby's diaper once breast milk starts flowing. Pink crystals should only be cause for concern if they persist beyond the first few days of life.

Do Babies Menstruate?

Kind of. It is normal for newborn girls to bleed from the vagina for a couple of days after birth. Babies are exposed to maternal hormones (i.e., estrogen) for nine months in the womb. After birth, the absence of hormonal exposure causes withdrawal bleeding similar to what is seen in menstruating adult women. Interestingly, maternal hormone exposure can also cause newborns (even boys!) to make breast milk for a few days.

Bottom Line: If you see the color red in your baby's diaper in the first few days after birth, consider some of the non-poo-related causes of bleeding discussed here. Once your kid starts eating regular food, remember to track everything he ate in the previous twenty-four hours. If no beets, Froot Loops, or red food coloring was consumed, you should march immediately to your pediatrician's office, red diaper in hand.

Steps to Survive Travel

As the world gets flatter, families become more spread out and family travel becomes more prevalent. When planning for your next trip, it's critical to be prepared. Unplanned bathroom stops are to be expected. Blowouts are inevitable. The following are some survival tips to help you prepare for your next family outing.

- Bring at least two easily accessible extra sets of clothes for your child. Three extra sets if the trip is longer than five hours. The clothes don't take up much space, and the costs of being unprepared are high.
- Bring one change of clothes for you, too. *Just in case.*
- Road trips: While iPads have made eight-hour car rides more tolerable for our children than they were when we were growing up, nature's call hasn't changed. Here are some tips:

- If your child is recently potty trained or in the midst of potty training, bring a plastic potty with you. You will have the flexibility of using it at the side of the road (and not praying your child can hold it until the next rest area, which is forty-six miles away). You may also need to use it if the public restrooms are in bad shape.

- Men's public restrooms are typically a lot more unpleasant than women's bathrooms, and unfortunately (or fortunately, depending on your perspective) often lack changing tables. On a road trip, it may be best for everyone if Mom takes charge of bathroom duty.

- Airplane rides: The honeymoon's over and so are the days of packing light and rolling aboard with your carry-on. You will now be lugging around multiple suitcases filled with diapers, extra wipes, maybe even a Pack 'n

Play. The key to survival is making sure to pack diapering essentials in your easily accessible carry-on bag.

- Airplane bathrooms felt cramped even before you had a kid. Now imagine you plus a thrashing baby in that minuscule

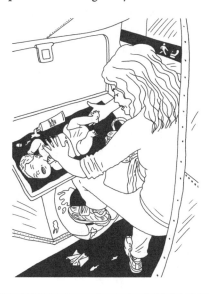

closet-like commode. Your child will inevitably try to touch everything in there and will almost certainly be too big for the changing table (it's more like a balance beam). You may want to consider changing your baby at your seat, especially if you and your spouse can set up walls on either side. The tray table is a last resort (please cover the table beforehand for sanitary reasons).

- If you attempt an in-your-seat diaper change, make sure to quickly contain the poopy diaper and wipes in a plastic bag. Otherwise, get ready for some unhappy neighbors as your child's poo aroma wafts throughout the recirculated cabin air.

A good parent's motto: Better to ask for forgiveness than to ask for permission.

Five

Baby Poo

Diarrhea

The runs, the Hershey Highway . . . whatever you call it—diarrhea is no fun. Feeling comfortable changing a poopy diaper? Proud that you can actually do this while also talking on the phone? Wait until you are elbow-deep in your little squirt's squirts before you anoint yourself the Diaper-Changing Champ.

Not only more difficult to contain than solid poo, diarrheal cleanup poses the added risk of you becoming sick. Most baby diarrhea is caused by a viral infection—rotavirus and norovirus being the two most common culprits. As you clean soiled diaper after soiled diaper, you put yourself at risk for contracting the very same infection. You must not only quickly and expertly change your kid's diaper in order to avoid catastrophe (Poonami, page 78), but you must do so in a way that keeps infectious organisms out of your own body.

The primary concern, of course, is for your baby's

health. The good news is that most diarrhea in kids is self-limited, meaning in a day or two the flow of diarrhea starts to resolve by itself. The most important part of treating viral GI infections, especially if vomiting is also involved, is to make sure your child doesn't become dehydrated.

The best way to know your baby is well hydrated is to keep track of the number of wet diapers. If your child is dehydrated, he won't be peeing as much. Assessing urine output can be difficult, however, if your child's diaper is always filled with liquid diarrhea.

Here are some other ways to tell your kid is down on fluids:

- Dry mouth
- Decreased tear production when crying
- Your kid looks lethargic, less active

Baby Gatorade

Use of an oral rehydration solution (ORS) is the best way to prevent and treat dehydration. The combination of electrolytes and glucose found in these drinks is similar to the composition of adult sports drinks, like Gatorade, absent the food coloring. Most children can be treated at home with oral solutions like Pedialyte until the diarrhea resolves and normal diet can resume. Flavored Pedialtye Popsicles work particularly well because, well, what kid doesn't like Popsicles? They also prevent kids from gulping down a lot of fluid at once (which can cause vomiting). Worldwide, the use of ORS in developing countries has dramatically reduced infant deaths due to diarrheal illnesses.

It's All in the Delivery, Baby

How a baby comes into this world has significant implications for how stool comes out. To review what many of us learned in eighth-grade health class—babies can be born one of two ways: through the vagina or via Cesarean section (C-section).

Some refer to vaginal deliveries as "natural" childbirth, meaning (we suppose) the way women were intended to deliver their babies. At times, however, this approach may jeopardize the baby's or mother's health, and a surgical approach, known as a C-section, is needed to remove the baby through the uterus after making an incision in the abdominal wall.

Whether a baby is delivered vaginally or via C-section will determine how much exposure the baby gets to Mom's bacteria. One of the benefits of a vaginal delivery is that babies ingest billions and billions of bacteria as they pass through the vaginal canal (yes, you read that correctly). Babies delivered via C-section, on the other hand, come into this world without such exposure to bacteria.

We have grown accustomed to thinking that bacteria are to be avoided ("Wash your hands!" "Cook your meat well!"). Turns out that this is one instance where being exposed to bacterial pathogens is a good thing. In fact, a robust bacterial inoculation is one of the best gifts a mother can give her newborn (aside from giving life and nourishment, of course).

Kids born vaginally tend to have fewer food allergies and less eczema than those born via C-section. In fact, allergic diseases are less common in kids whose parents used their saliva, which is chock-full of bacteria, to clean dirty pacifiers.

Bacterial exposure at the beginning of life is also vital to the development of the gastrointestinal tract. It prevents development of a serious intestinal condition called necrotizing enterocolitis, or NEC, for short. NEC affects premature babies and causes fever and abdominal swelling and can require surgery if severe.

Given the benefits of early exposure to bacteria, hospitals are now using probiotics, supplements of live, healthy bacteria, to prevent NEC

in high-risk babies. The theory is that by feeding babies healthy bacteria we can simulate the
natural exposure to bacteria that is vital to the
development of healthy digestive and immune
systems.

Poonami

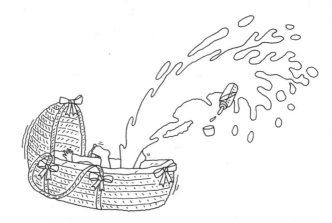

Hidden among the many rude awakenings of parenthood is the lesser known, but equally hazardous, Poonami. While diaper technology has improved over the decades, the Poonami continues to wreak havoc in newborn households all over the world.

Cleaning a diaper bogged down with acidic, watery

diarrhea is hard enough. Trying to control the carnage when there is more stool *outside* than inside the confines of the diaper is near impossible. Battle-tested parents can experience a PTSD-type reaction at the mere mention of the term *Poonami* (think of Striker as he tries to fly the plane with rivers of sweat pouring down his face in the movie *Airplane*).

The Poonami is a torrential elimination of liquid stool that can't be contained by a diaper and explodes up the baby's back. It tends to strike in the first few months of life, when baby poo is loose and expelled at high pressure along with intestinal gas. Poonamis run from the butt, up the spine, and can, in severe cases, reach the level of the shoulder blades. In the most severe cases, a Poonami can lead to fecal matter in the baby's hair. Ill-fitting diapers can also spring leaks through the thigh holes, causing a downward-trending Poonami involving one or both legs. Poonamis are trouble.

Early identification of a Poonami is crucial. There is nothing worse than laying down a baby with a backside blowout on the changing pad, which mercilessly spreads the collateral damage. Once the Poonami has been identified, all attempts to change the diaper on the changing pad should be quickly aborted. Head straight for the nearest source of running water (hose, sink faucet, etc.) and get to work. Baby wipes are only helpful if you are somehow able to hold your child upright with one arm while wiping his back in a downward direction with the other.

New parents often fall victim to the Poonami because of their reluctance to apply diapers snugly for fear of causing discomfort. Loosely applied diapers are a sure setup for liquid stool escape.

Just like other natural disasters, Poonamis have a classification system:

Class I: Minor spread of poo beyond the limits of the diaper.

Class II: Like a bubbling cauldron, the poo oozes beyond the diaper border, extends halfway up the back and/or halfway down the thighs, and the changing pad experiences contamination.

Class III: Widespread soilage that alters the color and feel of the baby's clothing, with evidence of the disaster also noticeable in the baby's hair and/or on the parent's clothing.

Bottom Line: Baby blowouts are inevitable and universal. The combination of liquid poo and intestinal gas makes it quite normal for infants to have explosive, liquid bowel movements in the first few months of life. Prevention is best attempted by applying diapers in a snug fashion. Poonami early detection is the key to an efficient cleanup, thereby minimizing the damage these natural disasters can create.

Diaper Rash

Changing a poopy diaper while your child is crying and violently thrashing can turn this already unpleasant chore into a nightmare. A common cause of a tormented diaper change is the presence of a diaper rash. This condition, also known as *dermatitis,* causes a fiery red rash affecting the buttocks and inner thighs. Diaper rashes cause significant pain and burning, especially when covered by urine and stool. Wiping this area during a diaper change is particularly painful, resulting in a fussy and unhappy baby.

Most diaper rashes occur because of prolonged buttock contact with pee or poo. These rashes are red, typically flat, and look like a really bad sunburn. The rashes occur in babies who have diarrhea or are sitting in a wet diaper for prolonged periods of time.

Diaper rashes can also occur with the introduction of new foods, the use of antibiotics, and changes in a breast-feeding mother's diet. Plastic diaper covers, while great for preventing stool leakage, trap moisture near your baby's skin, increasing the risk of getting a diaper rash, and are generally not recommended.

Treatment for mild cases of diaper rash starts with changing your baby's diaper frequently. Drying the buttocks before placing on a clean diaper can also help (Russian Poolette, page 86). Petroleum jelly and lanolin are good preventive measures, especially at night when babies have prolonged exposure to a wet diaper. Zinc oxide is the mainstay for treatment once the rash has developed.

Avoid using scented wipes or perfumed lotions, which may further irritate your baby's skin. Also, don't use talcum powder. This age-old treatment can cause lung problems in kids if the powder is inhaled.

Occasionally, a diaper rash may be caused

by a fungal infection. This rash is also red but, unlike the typical flat diaper rash, appears beefy and raised. Fungi thrive in dark, moist areas like those cute baby thigh folds. Treatment requires a topical antifungal cream in addition to the measures discussed above.

Bottom Line: Rest assured that you are not expected to be a dermatologist. If the rash doesn't get better with simple measures, talk to your pediatrician.

Petroleum Jelly

To many, petroleum jelly is a magic elixir. If you need to survive on a desert island with your baby and can bring only one toiletry with you, this may be it. It can be used for diaper rash and protection for scrapes, as well as a cure for chapped lips. While it can cure many maladies, it may be best to dedicate a jar just for your baby's bum, and a separate one for lips and scrapes. This way, you can avoid the inadvertent double doo-doo dip—that is, applying poo-soiled petroleum jelly to other parts of your (or your baby's) body.

Russian Poolette

A particularly effective (and bold) strategy to relieve diaper rash is to allow your child "air time," that is, time without a diaper. Leaving the diaper off keeps the skin dry and can hasten recovery from a diaper rash. If you decide to let your baby air it out, however, be forewarned that you are engaging in a dangerous game of Russian Poolette.

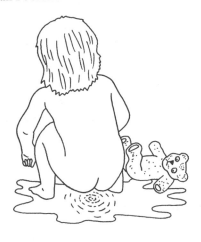

After seeing a fiery red rash during a diaper change, a parent may decide that the wise move is to let Junior roam free and delay application of a new diaper for a few hours. The upside of this strategy is that it can lead to a drier, and certainly happier, baby. Even kids without diaper rashes experience a sense of liberation from being in their natural, naked state.

The downside of a kid who is not potty trained running around in his birthday suit should be obvious— pee and poo carpet bombing.

Bottom Line: There is no question, allowing your child some air time is an effective treatment for a diaper rash. But are you willing to pay the price? Kids not yet potty trained will pee or poo when they feel like it. Air time is an ill-advised, high-risk, low-reward game, particularly in kids with diarrhea (for obvious reasons).

The Grain Drain

The introduction of solid foods can be an exciting yet difficult time. Feedings are messier and take longer than the good ol' days of breast- and bottle-feeding. The introduction of food choices adds a whole new complexity to providing nourishment to your child.

Babies may have ever-changing preferences for food tastes and textures, which make finding the right menu challenging. While some kids are more finicky than others, some of this pain is self-inflicted by parents. Take, for instance, the universal practice of forcing a child to consume mashed green beans. One whiff of the nauseating aroma coming from the baby food jar should be enough to know that this force-feeding is not going to end well.

Another challenge of the solid food era can occur at age six months with the introduction of wheat-based cereals. (Iron-fortified cereals are needed around this time because babies' iron stores from Mom have been depleted.) The onset of diarrhea, abdominal discomfort, gas, and failure to appropriately gain weight can all be signs of a condition called celiac disease.

Celiac disease is an intestinal disorder caused by an inability to correctly digest gluten, a common ingredient found in foods made of wheat, rye, and barley. This results in damage to the intestinal lining, causing diarrhea and difficulty absorbing nutrients.

Bottom Line: You should think about getting your baby tested for celiac disease if there is a family history of this condition or your child begins exhibiting symptoms of diarrhea or poor weight gain after transitioning to solid foods. Blood tests can determine if your child is at risk for celiac disease, and can help guide dietary changes.

Breast milk may protect babies from developing celiac disease. Research has shown that infants who were breast-feeding at the time they were introduced to gluten-containing foods (around six months of age) were less likely to develop celiac disease then those who were formula-fed. One theory points to the beneficial effects of *Bifidobacterium*, a healthy bacterium found in breast milk. Exposure to this bacterium quiets down a baby's immune system, making it less likely to adversely react to gluten molecules.

The Refill, aka the Double Down

Free refills aren't always a good thing.

Babies have this uncanny knack of unleashing more poo just as you slap down a clean diaper. This bizarre, yet ubiquitous, phenomenon (also known as doubling down) tends to play out like this:

Junior is acting fussy and the stench you have come to know all too well is emanating from his diaper. You trudge upstairs and lay him down on the changing pad, ready to make quick work of this cleanup. As you finish the job and seal up his clean diaper, you hear the Grunt (page 94) and catch him making his characteristic poopy face. *You've got to be kidding me,* you think.

Before you can react, round two has been deployed. If you are lucky, the new diaper has been applied and the goods have landed in the diaper. If not, get ready to scoop the deposit off the changing pad and explain

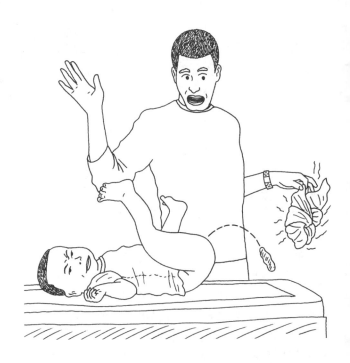

to your spouse why the plush, powder-blue changing pad is now streaked with brown skid marks.

What is it about fresh air and a clean diaper that stimulates another bowel movement? At times, eager parents will change a dirty diaper too soon, not allowing for complete evacuation. It is usually a good idea to wait a few extra minutes after you first smell a bowel movement to make sure your li'l one is done with the deed.

The Refill most commonly occurs while changing a diaper after a meal. Eating stimulates the intestines to push things downstream and may cause back-to-back BMs. Others have claimed that there is something calming, and natural, about being unconstrained by a diaper. This feeling of relaxation stimulates the bowels to move, similar to what adults experience when we are in·our home bathroom, reading our favorite magazine (*Lock and Load!*).

Bottom Line: When it comes to the Refill, you must acknowledge its unpredictability. Always be prepared. Minimize "air time," that is, the time your baby's backside is exposed to air, by readying the new diaper before you remove the old one. This will save you the agony of cleaning the changing pad and, more important, prevent rebuke from your significant other.

The Grunt

If you thought you hated former tennis star Monica Seles's grunting during every stroke, wait till you grow familiar with the cacophony of your child's poo grunt. Sure, at first listen, there is nothing harsh about this sound. In fact, it's not even that loud. To be true, it's not even the sound itself. It's what comes next.

The Grunt is often accompanied by the Look (a countenance that can only be described as a mixture of concentration and straining). Both are signs of an impending need to change a dirty, smelly diaper. Your body will instantly react with a faint sense of nausea, even mild perspiration, as you subconsciously recall the pain associated with previous Grunts. Who can forget the Grunt just before that monstrous bowel movement during that long drive to visit your mother-in-law? Or the one that seems to happen every night at 3 AM?

Why do babies grunt when they poop? *You try having a bowel movement while lying on your back.* The combination of poor positioning (which is no fault of their own) and weak abdominal muscles means your little one has to push extra hard in order to generate the force needed to expel stool.

There *is* a way to use the Grunt to your advantage. Let's say you are cuddled up with your child, watching your favorite TV program, while your husband is "working" in the office. Your child flashes the Look and makes a few usual noises signaling to you that it is about time for a diaper change. At this instant, you quickly yell to your husband that you forgot to take out the trash and ask if *he can keep an eye on Junior*. Imagine his surprise when, a few minutes later, he is overcome with the smell of a dirty diaper and proceeds to change it.

This, my friends, is what we call a perfect *poopy trap*.

Don't Take a Stand

Every parent, once their child is old enough to stand, will attempt to change a diaper with their child in the upright position. Whether you undertake this challenge to test your skills or you think it's the easiest way to change a baby on the go, the upright diaper change is a bad idea (most of us learn the hard way).

We may resort to the standing diaper change because of a forgotten changing pad or to avoid a dirty, unhygienic floor. The inevitable result is a loosely, asymmetrically applied diaper that will either (a) slide off your baby's butt, or (b) spring a leak. The worst-case scenario occurs during removal of the dirty diaper when you realize, a little too late, that what you thought was a wet diaper actually contains poo. You are now confronted with a standing child (who can possibly run away) with feces smeared on his butt and thighs. If he really does make a break for it, God help you.

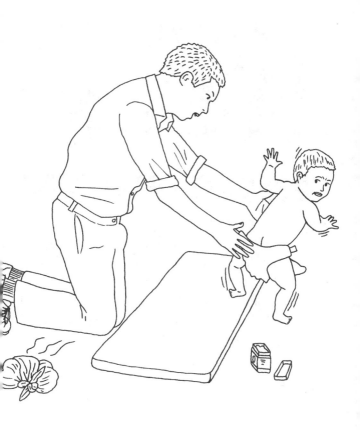

Heed the advice (you probably won't) to never change a diaper while your baby is standing. At the very least, employ the Dipstick maneuver (see below) to make sure you're not dealing with poo.

Dipstick

It's sometimes hard to determine whether or not your child needs a diaper change. The typical technique is to pick Junior up, put his butt up against your nose, and take a big whiff. While that often works, it's far from foolproof (and frankly, not much fun). Sometimes a parent has a cold. Other times, poo may be odorless. When you suspect the need for a diaper change but your sense of smell doesn't provide a definitive answer, it's time to engage your other senses.

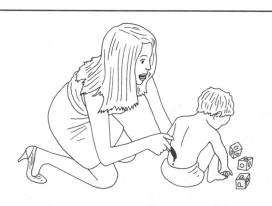

In the case of a wet diaper, the telltale diaper sag can alert you to the need for a change. When poo is in question, some parents will utilize the Dipstick technique. This maneuver involves curling a finger around the diaper's back edge in order to peek inside and see if there's any poop. While effective, this technique is fraught with perils. An overly aggressive finger insertion during the diaper pullback can lead to an unexpected, and unwanted, surprise.

Survival Tip

Unlike when you're eating chocolate fondue, you never want to end up with a brown finger during a diaper Dipstick. It is safer to peek in from the top of the back of the diaper while your child is in the upright position rather than pull back the elastic around the thighs. Remember, poo doesn't defy gravity and is usually sitting at the bottom of the diaper.

Toothy Poo

A baby's first tooth is considered to be an important milestone, one to cherish and jot down in that baby journal next to the first time your little one rolled over on his own. While noteworthy, the appearance of the first tooth is not all smiles and giggles.

The first tooth usually appears between four and six months of age (sometimes later) and is preceded by days or weeks of fussiness, poor sleeping, torrential drooling, and a decreased desire to feed. To top things off, the GI tract goes haywire and begins pumping out a landslide of loose, mushy stool. This diarrhea begins a few days before the first tooth appears and can even be accompanied by a low-grade fever. Initially, this combination of symptoms in a fussy child is often incorrectly attributed to a viral infection. Your child's day-care provider may grow tired of changing diaper after diaper and call you to take your incessantly poop-ing child to the doctor.

What does a baby's first tooth have to do with poop? Well, it turns out nobody is really sure. All we know is that this unique form of diarrhea can be the first sign that the teething era (and all the joy it brings) is upon you.

A possible cause of diarrhea is the massive saliva load. One of the classic signs of a teething kid (other than her chomping on your fingers any chance she gets) is the waterfall of drool emerging from her mouth. Since most of this excessive drool is swallowed, it may tax a baby's immature intestines to the point where it causes loose stools.

Bottom Line: Recognizing that short-lived diarrhea can be associated with your baby's first tooth will prevent unnecessary worry (and hopefully keep your child in day care). Diarrhea usually resolves just as the first tooth begins to rear its ugly, uh, beautiful head.

The Deuce Is Loose

(A) That's Not a Baby
Ruth in the Pool

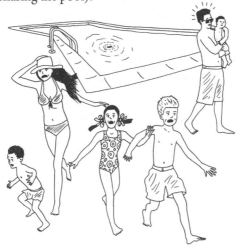

Swim diapers make taking your baby to the pool a much more pleasurable experience. They provide a level of comfort both for the parent and for the baby who isn't yet potty trained (not to mention the other people sharing the pool).

The absorbency in standard diapers comes from sodium polyacrylate crystals that soak up urine and help keep your baby dry. Just as in Monty Python's *The Meaning of Life*, when a wafer-thin mint causes the morbidly obese Mr. Creosote to explode, even the most absorbent diapers can burst if soaked in enough liquid. Swim diapers, however, obviate this problem by allowing urine to exit the diaper while retaining (more harmful) solid waste.

Some parents will forgo the swim diaper and take their baby in the pool au naturel. This is a risky proposition for you and anyone else who may swim in that pool, and is fortunately against the rules at most public pools.

If your baby happens to unleash a pool poo, aka a chockodile, fast action is required.

1. Get your child and everyone else out of the pool.
2. If you have already been identified as the parent whose kid pooped in the pool, you might as well try to remove the poop before it

spreads. This will limit its detrimental effects and maybe encourage people to forgive you. Removal with a nearby towel or cup should only be attempted if the stool is solid.

3. In the unfortunate event that your child has diarrhea, cleanup is not possible (think *Exxon Valdez*). Our only advice in this scenario is to notify the authorities and quickly pack up and leave the premises.

The typical response to a loose deuce in the pool is to "shock" the water by spiking chlorine levels to kill off all of the fecal bacteria. In the case of explosive diarrhea, a more comprehensive cleaning is required. The Centers for Disease Control has clear guidelines on recommended chlorine levels and times in between poo cleanup and safe return to swimming.

Bottom Line: Unless you are 100 percent sure your child won't poop in the pool . . . don't be that guy. Have him wear a swim diaper. Consider skipping the pool altogether if Junior has been having loose stools.

Even the best swim diapers can't keep diarrhea out of the pool.

Survival Tip

Don't put on the swim diaper until you get to the pool. The swim diaper is designed to contain poop, not to soak up liquid. If your child is strapped into the car seat wearing a swim diaper, be prepared to find a pool of your own in the backseat of your car.

If a Tree Falls in the Woods and Nobody Is Around, Does It Make a Sound?

If you and your child are the only two people in the pool at the time of the poo, it may present a moral dilemma for you as a parent. The response to poo in a pool is to close, clean, and maybe even drain the pool before refilling it with fresh water (think of the movie *Caddyshack* and the response to the floating Baby Ruth). This represents a lot of work, cost, and inconvenience, and can be particularly embarrassing if you're the reason the community pool has to close on a hot summer day.

So after you scoop out the poop, what do you do if nobody else saw it happen? While it may be embarrassing, you have a moral obligation to notify the pool management and make sure you don't cause a massive giardia or E. coli outbreak.

(B) That's Not a Baby
Ruth in the Tub

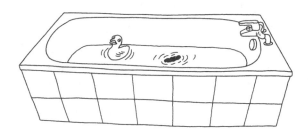

Until babies are potty trained, they will relieve themselves wherever and whenever nature calls. While this freedom to poo or pee at any moment is not a problem for parents when their child is wearing a diaper, waste cleanup suddenly becomes problematic when your li'l one is in a bathtub. The difficulties increase exponentially when your baby is sharing the bath with a sibling, friend, or, even worse, you.

So what do you do when your child's joyful bath time suddenly darkens due to the presence of poo? First, rest assured that the appearance of this new "toy" in the tub is not too uncommon. While quickly removing all children from the bath is paramount, the consistency of the poo will help dictate how dire your dilemma is.

Chockodile: In the case of a solid poo, whether pebble-sized or larger, floater or sinker, it is easy to isolate the transgression. Assuming you remove your child before he turns his bowel movement into his new rubber ducky, cleanup can be fairly simple. See the survival tips on page 111.

Exxon Valdez: Bath-time diarrhea is another one of parenthood's true emergencies. The management of solid poo will seem like child's play compared to this natural disaster. With solid poo you have the option of removing the waste quickly and then removing your child (although we always recommend baby removal first). When the accident takes on a liquid form, the *only* correct first step is to rescue your child before he is consumed by this oil slick.

The other challenge posed by diarrhea in the tub is the uncertainty of whether there is more to come. We recommend placing your baby in an empty sink or holding him perched on the toilet until you are sure the river has run dry. This will obviously delay cleanup efforts, but the last thing you want is a poopy trail all over your bathroom.

Can poo in the tub be a good thing? Turns out it can. A common remedy for a constipated baby is to place them in a tub of warm water. This can relax muscles and make kids more inclined to unleash a hard bowel movement.

If you go this route (we think prune juice is easier), just be prepared to quickly extract your baby and then the poo, which thankfully will be hard in consistency, as soon as the deed is done.

Steps to Surviving the Unwelcome Poo in the Tub

1. Call for help if your spouse or any other adult is around. This is no time to be a hero.
2. Remove your child from the tub immediately. (Don't throw out the baby with the bathwater.)
3. Close the bathroom door to confine the situation to one room.
4. Call for help again if help hasn't yet arrived.
5. If you successfully remove your child before any significant contact with stool, skip to step 8.
6. If your child picks up the poo to start playing with it, be sure to *thoroughly* clean her hands with soap.
7. If there is any chance that your child ingested poop, call your pediatrician.
8. Remove all of the toys from the tub. Quarantine them in a bucket, in the sink, or any-

where else out of reach of your child. Thoroughly clean them later (or throw them out), but don't think about that during this time of triage.

9. Take a cup and start scooping the poop out of the tub. Dump each turd into the toilet. Once a cup is used for poop removal, we recommend that you no longer use it for bath time (or drinking) in the future.

10. Drain the tub.

11. If you have a bath mat in the tub, be sure to remove that and clean it separately. . . . Poo particles can get trapped between the tub and the mat.

12. Thoroughly rinse the tub and the bath mat with a rag. Bleach is a good thing.

13. It's time to finish bath time. We recommend using a different bathtub.

Giardia

There's diarrhea and there's *diarrhea*. *Giardia lamblia* infection is like the customary viral gastroenteritis on steroids. First, this protozoal infection causes an unmistakably abhorrent odor. In water, these stools classically float on the surface of the toilet; in a diaper, the diarrhea takes on a foamy appearance. Throw in the agony of rampant gas production and you have one unhappy baby (and family).

Humans become infected by drinking contaminated water from lakes, wells, etc., and then pass it on to others through poor hygiene practices. Infants shouldn't be drinking water (or ingesting lake water, for that matter) but can become infected while at day care. Though unpleasant, the good news is that a *Giardia* infection usually resolves in a few days. Antibiotics can hasten recovery and prevent chronic infection, which can lead to poor nutrition and growth.

Dairy Doo

Milk. It does a body good. And those milk mustaches are so cute! But can too much milk be a bad thing? Turns out the answer is yes.

Many an overzealous parent has force-fed their youngster bottle upon bottle of milk in hopes of churning out the next Shaquille O'Neal. Frankly, milk seems like the best option when you consider the cautions against fruit juice (and most kids don't want to drink water). Milk has become a nutritional staple in the industrialized world, a means to raising strong, healthy kids.

A moderate amount of milk (maximum 24 ounces a day) introduced after one year of age is important for brain development. The high fat content in whole milk is helpful for central nervous system myelination (myelin is nerve insulation that allows brain signals to be conducted rapidly). After age two, brain development slows and most pediatricians recommend switching to low-fat milk.

In addition to being a good source of protein, cow's milk is rich in calcium and vitamin D, two nutrients that are crucial for bone growth. Soy milk packs a similar nutritional punch and can be used in cases where cow's milk is not desired or feasible (due to allergies, for example).

Despite the long list of benefits, early introduction of cow's milk can have its downsides, particularly when it comes to a baby's gastrointestinal tract.

The most alarming drawback of milk is its potential for causing anemia, or low red blood cell counts. Kids can also develop a milk-protein allergy where diarrhea and blood-streaked stools are the end result. In susceptible kids, the intestinal lining becomes inflamed when it comes in contact with the proteins found in cow's milk.

Interestingly, this milk-protein allergy can rear its head even while kids are being breast-fed exclusively. Cow's milk proteins consumed by the mother find their way into breast milk and are ingested by infants, eventually causing irritation to the baby's GI tract. In this scenario, breast-feeding can continue, but the mother must eliminate all dairy products from her diet.

Though infrequent, when this occurs, it means no milk in Mom's morning cup of coffee—another one of many painful sacrifices you will make for your kids.

Raw Deal

When it comes to food, organic has become synonymous with health. We don't want our meat injected with hormones and we don't want our beets grown in pesticide-laden soil. But does anyone really want raw, unpasteurized cow's milk for their baby? Yes. (*That rustling is the sound of Louis Pasteur turning in his grave.*)

Many parents believe in the benefits of raw milk and feed it to their kids. Raw milk propo-

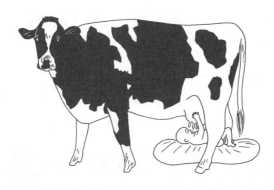

nents feel drinking unprocessed milk straight from the cow's teat leads to a stronger immune system and lowers the risk of environmental and food allergies. There is a burgeoning movement sweeping the nation, and feeding raw milk to your kid is legal in many states.

The problem with raw milk is, well, that it is *raw*. It does not undergo pasteurization, a process meant to decrease the transmission of infections from cows to humans. Concern about raw milk's safety spiked after reports of serious infections with E. coli and *Listeria* in young children consuming unpasteurized milk. Turns out good ol' Louis Pasteur was on to something when he figured out it is a good idea to sterilize milk before consumption.

Antibiotic Poo

Ear infections will happen to virtually all young children. Treatment is straightforward and often includes a course of antibiotics. While helpful to relieve ear pain and swelling, antibiotics can harm the GI tract, causing watery diarrhea for days or weeks at a time. Loose stools can continue even after the antibiotic course has been completed.

Antibiotics kill bacteria, both good and bad. Diarrhea results from the eradication of healthy bacteria residing in your baby's intestinal tract.

This affects the way they digest certain foods and, at times, can mimic a GI infection or food allergy. The good news is that symptoms will resolve in time. Recovery can be hastened by giving your kids pediatrician-approved probiotics to restore a healthy bacterial balance in your kid's intestinal tract.

Juicy Deuce

Technically called "toddler's diarrhea," the floodgates on this form of diarrhea tend to open up between one and three years of age and is the result of so-called high-carbohydrate beverages, known to us common folk as fruit juice.

Juice seems to be blamed for all childhood ills these days. Obesity, dental cavities, even ADHD. The way some moms talk about juice you would think it was crack cocaine. *(Can you believe Jake's mom? I heard she sent him to school with fruit punch in his sippy cup last week!)* Some moms have even been known to forbid playdates with kids who indulge in these artificially flavored and colored drinks.

When it comes to poo, the high concentration of simple sugars found in fruit juice can tax the digestive capabilities of the developing GI tract and cause loose, watery stools. At first, you may fear a viral gastroenteritis, but quick recognition of excessive intake of sugar-laden beverages can save you a trip to the doctor. Substitution of water and other unsweetened drinks can result in immediate cessation of the diarrhea.

An added benefit of going juice-free? More play-dates for your kid.

Poocasso

Children are curious. As a parent, it's your job to nurture your child's desire to explore and learn, and to foster creative expression. There are times, however, when curiosity and creativity go too far.

It is not uncommon for a parent to enter a child's room and see him awake in the crib with his or her pants and diaper off, smearing poop on the walls.

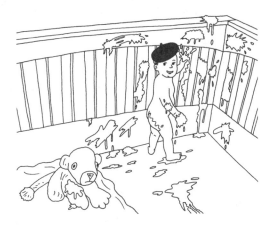

Don't blame yourself for not having adequate finger-painting supplies on hand. Kids will find inspiration *anywhere*.

Bottom Line: First and foremost, when encountering your child's Doodie Doodles, focus on the cleanup. After your child and her canvas have been sterilized, do not fret. It is perfectly normal for children around the age of two to begin to notice their feces and play with it. Remember that Picasso was once a baby, too.

How to Survive If Your Child Is an Aspiring Thomas Kinkade of Poop

While some children will dabble in finger painting with poop and then never do it again, other such artists will enter a prolonged "Brown Period" where poop becomes their preferred medium. While we hate to stifle creativity, repeatedly cleaning poop off the walls can get old, fast.

Some tactics to prevent future poo paintings:

- Apply duct tape or plastic wrap around the diaper.
- Put your baby to sleep in a onesie under her normal pj's.
- Put pj's on backward so that the snaps/zipper are on the back.

Despite these creative deterrents to diaper removal, babies still sometimes find a way to turn their poop into paint. Scolding a child for being curious about the warm excrement in his or her diaper likely won't accomplish much. So what is a parent to do?

When all attempts to prevent future artistic creations using feces fail, try subjecting her to a cold shower immediately upon discovering the poop smear. Pick your child up, calmly explain that poop needs to remain in the diaper or in the potty, then clean her off in a cold shower. While your child will scream and hate it, the association of playing with poop and a cold shower should reorient your child to resume using more traditional non-fecal art supplies again.

Seven-Month Itch

Sometimes when a baby is approximately seven months old, things get a bit, shall we say, interesting. Every chance he gets, especially at night while sleeping, Junior seems to be on a mission to tear off his diaper and scratch his backside. Is this fixation simply a manifestation of Freud's anal stage? Or just another quirk of babyhood?

Excessive nighttime itching is a classic sign of pinworm infection, one of the most common parasitic infections in the industrialized world. In children, pinworm infection runs rampant during the day-care/preschool years. Kids tend to have the irresistible urge to scratch their backsides when worms come out at night to lay eggs outside the anal canal (the eggs irritate the skin around the anus). After collecting these eggs on their hands, children spread them to others by touching toys and books.

If you aren't sufficiently grossed out yet, let's discuss how this diagnosis is often made. The infamous "Scotch tape test" will test any parent's devotion to their children. Prior to bedtime, a piece of Scotch tape is used to create a trap of sorts for these nocturnal worms when they exit the anal canal to lay their eggs. The tape is applied transversely between the buttocks (creating a bridge of sorts, sticky side facing in). The tape is removed in the morning and examined (yes, by the parents) for the culprit eggs.

Some (wise) parents will opt to forgo such testing and treat their child with antiparasitic medications when they notice this characteristic itch.

Sleep-Training Poo

Several months of no sleep is enough. You and your spouse decide it is time to sleep train your child. After consulting books and websites (and weighing the unsolicited advice of more "experienced" parents), you decide to adopt the seemingly cruel but effective "cry it out" method.

After several nights of caving in to the violent shrieking of your precious little one, you vow to really let her cry it out this time. Like clockwork, 3 AM comes and the siren goes off. As much as it pains you, you allow the crying to go on—five minutes, ten minutes. . . . You can picture her in the crib wailing, likely shaking with fear as you, parent and guardian, allow her to suffer. Fifteen minutes . . . twenty minutes . . .

That's it, you think. I can't take it. I'm going in.

As soon as you enter the room, your nose

alerts you to the harsh truth—a dirty diaper is to blame for this middle-of-the-night freak-out. You are overwhelmed with guilt. *What kind of parent would let their kid scream for almost a half hour while sitting in her own poop?!*

Bottom Line: Don't blame yourself. Sleep training is a harrowing time, and there is no way to know why your child is crying. Plus, there is little harm in allowing your child to remain with a poopy diaper for a few minutes. Plus, you need the sleep.

Snack Attack, aka Déjà Poo

With the introduction of solid foods comes the joy of the Snack Attack, also affectionately known as Déjà Poo. With the exception of seeds and curds, your child's breast milk and formula diet has resulted in poo with uniform consistency. Now that solids have been introduced, you are not sure what you'll find when you open your child's diaper.

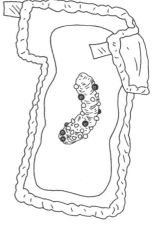

Most parents will never forget the first time they peel off a dirty diaper and see remnants of a prior meal mixed in with stool. Green peas, blueberries, and, of course, corn are the most common culprits. These items can fly through the GI tract and show up in a diaper in their original form a mere few hours after consumption.

It is only natural to wonder, "Is my child digesting properly?" "Am I feeding him too much?" These moments will have you longing for the good ol' days of smooth, brown poop.

Bottom Line: Foods high in insoluble fiber, like peas and corn, are not digested by the human digestive system and are supposed to come out looking the same way they went in. Déjà Poo occurs in adults and young children alike. Most important, seeing corn or a tomato skin in your child's poop does not mean there is anything wrong with your child's digestion. You can (and should) continue to feed your child these high-fiber foods. Just be ready for the aftermath. . . .

Baby Logjam

Parents of a newborn spend most of their waking lives obsessed with their child's poop. Even as they find creative ways to wiggle out of diaper changes, parents will discreetly keep tabs on their baby's poo scorecard. *Was it soft, honey? What color was it? How many does that make today, anyway?*

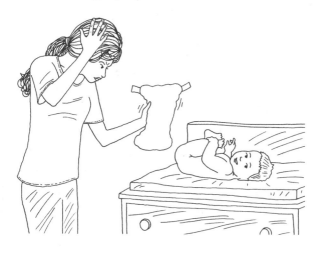

For some, newborn nutrition takes a backseat to their baby's back-door business. A new parent, returning from a day's work, is more apt to inquire about the number of dirty diapers than the number of adequate feedings. In the overwhelming world of new parenthood, when poo's steady stream slows down, all hell can break loose.

Just like with adults, what goes in strongly affects what comes out. Diet plays a big role in determining how many diapers your little one will blow through in a day. Most breast-fed babies will have a BM after every feeding (about six a day). Formula-feeders tip the scale at three or four a day.

Not having a bowel movement for a day or two does not mean your child is constipated. Stool consistency and a baby's disposition are better indicators of an impending plumbing problem. Hard or pellet-sized stool associated with grimacing, straining, and discomfort/fussiness are more concerning than a drop in the bowel movement tally (alas, it's not all about the numbers).

Most of the time, infants develop hard, particulate stools because of dietary changes or discomfort around the anal opening (it's no fun to have a bowel movement when your bum hurts). Your little one may decide to hold in stool because of soreness resulting from an anal fissure (a tear in the anal sphincter muscle) or a bad diaper rash.

Infants receiving iron-fortified and soy-based formulas and rice cereal can develop hard, pebble-like poo. Because babies need this extra iron, you should try to continue these iron-fortified formulas and manage constipation after consulting with your pediatrician. A teaspoon or so of diluted prune juice with feedings usually does the trick. Water can be given but in very limited amounts (an ounce or two at most) after checking with your baby's pediatrician (a newborn baby's kidneys can't process larger quantities).

Rectal stimulation with a rectal thermometer or suppository should be reserved for severe cases (inflicting more pain on your child who is already uncomfortable can be counterproductive). Plus, babies can become dependent on rectal stimulation if used too often.

Poo Paradox

When does diarrhea = constipation? In a condition known as overflow diarrhea. Extreme constipation can lead to fecal impaction, essentially a stool plug that blocks the passage of solid stool. In severe cases, liquid stool can leak around the edges of the impacted stool plug and come out looking like diarrhea. Liquid bowel movements can fool parents into thinking that their child is having diarrhea when the real problem is constipation. In reality, the amount of liquid stool is much smaller than would be expected in cases of, say, infectious diarrhea. Finding your child straining and grunting during loose bowel movements can be clues that you are dealing with a Poo Paradox. Treatment of constipation will resolve this unusual cause of "diarrhea."

Poo Protest

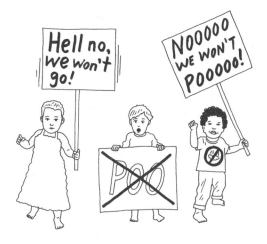

Babies have minds of their own. Even before they can talk they have a way of making their feelings known. Take, for example, the very common act of throwing unsavory food items on the floor. This assertiveness applies to the world of poo as well.

For reasons that are not altogether clear, babies have the penchant for withholding poo when they are unsettled by their surroundings. It is common for infants not to poop for days at a time while traveling or when a parent or primary caretaker is away. This is rarely a cause for concern. In fact, while in the midst of a poo protest, babies seem just fine and rarely exhibit any signs of distress. The protest will end just as quickly as it began when the baby regains a sense of comfort and security.

At first glance, the poo protest may seem like odd behavior, but we have long known that babies (and adults, for that matter) tend to go more often and freely when they are in a soothing environment. For adults, this typically means being in a familiar bathroom, reading a good magazine or playing our favorite iPad game. For toddlers, seeking comfort may manifest itself in a quick dart to a quiet, private corner.

A more severe form of poo protest, known as encopresis, is seen in older children as they reach potty-training age. This repeated, volitional holding of stool is a concerning behavioral problem requiring medical attention.

The poo protest is typically a manifestation of what

happens when babies cannot create the inner and outer sanctuary needed to freely have a bowel movement. Evolutionarily, withholding poo in strange environments may have aided survival (poo is commonly used as a way for predatory animals to track their prey).

When a prolonged poo protest ends, beware the potential for an impending Poonami or monster poo!

Poo Envy

If you haven't experienced parental poo envy yet, you will. You will never forget the first time your child runs out of the bathroom yelling, "Daddy, you've gotta see the size of this!" One of parenthood's most unexpected moments occurs on the day you peer into the toilet bowl or into a full diaper and grow envious of your child's bowel movement. Yes, you read correctly. Whether it takes three months or three years, there will come a day in the not-so-distant future when you wish you could manufacture solid waste like your child.

We can all imagine our children being able to run faster and jump higher than we can. There may even come a day when they grow smarter. But is it humanly possible for a small child to produce a bowel movement that is larger than an adult's? The harsh reality is that this is not only possible, it is a virtual certainty.

We affectionately refer to particularly large evacua-

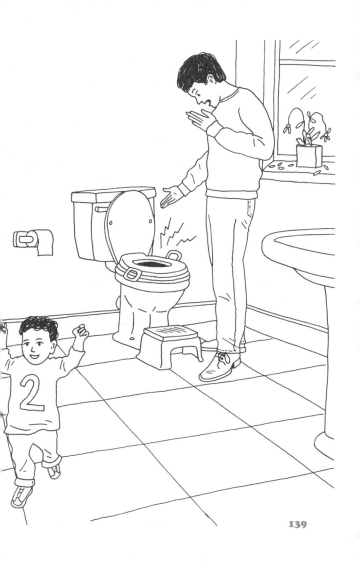

139

tions as *monster poos*. These sizable bowel movements are created by a robust dietary intake of fiber and water (picture the engorgement of beans soaking in water).

Infants and toddlers tend to eat high-fiber diets (because we feed them healthy foods like fresh fruits and vegetables) while we consume pizza and burgers. Further, a young intestinal tract is the model of efficiency while many adult colons have become lazy due to medications, poor diet, and general social constraints (we can't exactly go to the bathroom whenever we feel like it). The longer we hold on to stool, the harder and more constipated our bowels.

We will learn a lot from our children. Among these early lessons is the importance of healthy bowel habits.

Six

Pee, Vomit, and Gas

Pee Palette

If the Poo Palette is paint, the Pee Palette is watercolor.

Ninety-nine percent of baby pee will be some shade of yellow, identified primarily by the color of the diaper stain. While not as varied as poo, pee color can also be an important indicator of baby health.

Yellow

The normal yellow color of urine is caused by the presence of urobilinogen, a by-product of bile. The higher the urobilinogen concentration, the darker the shade of yellow, which can be a warning sign of dehydration.

Because babies can't tell you when they are thirsty, urine color becomes an important marker of their hydration status. Early in life, dark yellow pee means your child is not getting enough breast milk or formula. The ideal color is that of pale lemonade, almost clear but tinged with a hint of yellow.

Red

In the first few days of life, mild dehydration in a newborn can lead to formation of uric acid crystals. This can show up in the diaper looking like a red stain or, with closer inspection, red powdery debris. This is not cause for concern and should resolve as your baby begins breast-feeding.

The other common cause of red urine in young children is a urinary tract infection, in either the bladder or the kidneys. Fever, fussiness, and foul-smelling urine can be clues that an infection is to blame.

For older kids, remember that just like beets can turn poo red, they can have a similar impact on children's pee!

Brown

Persistently brown, Coca-Cola–colored urine can be a sign of a bile blockage, usually due to a problem with the liver or bile ducts. Dark-colored urine is usually seen in tandem with light-colored stool (the bile "backs up" into the urine instead of being mixed with the stool).

Fountain of Youth

Congratulations, Dad. It's a boy!

You dream of days in the park, playing catch, and Sunday afternoons watching football (and you finally have someone else to mow the lawn). Before any of that, though, it's your turn to change the diaper.

You pick up your li'l all-star and take a quick sniff

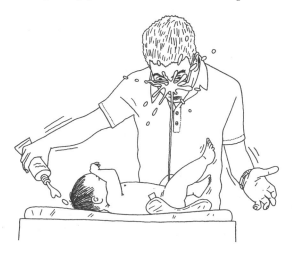

to assess the damage. It's your lucky day—no smell means no poo. Eager to obtain credit for an easy diaper change, you yell out to your wife, "Don't worry, honey, I got this one."

After laying down your bundle of joy (you must admit, he *is* cute), you proceed to confidently tear off the soggy, urine-laden diaper with one hand while reaching for a baby wipe with the other. Proud of your quick mastery of fatherhood, you are brought back to reality as a warm stream of fluid splatters onto the side of your face. You wonder if the roof has sprung another leak.

Alas, no. Welcome to fatherhood. You have just been struck by your son's golden Fountain of Youth. Unfortunately, this Fountain of Youth won't restore you to a younger age (although urine *is* good for your skin).

Many a new parent has been victimized by the Fountain of Youth. Like an untethered, fully open garden hose flailing wildly in the yard, male newborns have little control over where their urine stream ends up. They also have this knack for letting loose at exactly the wrong time. Some have theorized that the open air stimulates the urge to urinate, while others believe this is just another inexplicable newborn quirk designed to further torment new parents.

Either way, good diapering technique can minimize the collateral damage. First, make sure to minimize air time by preparing the new diaper before removing the old one. The "tuck technique" is also crucial to prevent the urine stream from flying through the air. This method involves redirecting your son's hose so it is pointing down, ideally into the awaiting fresh diaper.

Can't wait until li'l John starts using the toilet? Be careful what you wish for. In a few years you will be cleaning up poorly aimed urine from places you never thought possible.

Pee-Pee Teepee

When changing Junior, traditional thinking dictates that speed is crucial in order to avoid getting hit by the Fountain of Youth. Utilizing the Pee-Pee Teepee, however, allows for a more relaxed diaper change. The teepee technique involves placing a cone or cup over Junior's johnson immediately after taking off the old diaper. This strategy won't prevent your baby from peeing with the diaper off, but it will save you from a most unwanted golden shower courtesy of your baby boy.

Beware the Baby Boner

A baby erection is one of the most shocking moments for any parent (probably more so for moms). The baby boner is almost always discovered during a diaper change (there must be something about being free and loose) and can seem unnatural. Rest assured that this is a completely normal physiologic process, even if your child is only a few weeks old. Infant erections are *not* caused by an Oedipal complex (it's too soon for that).

While this information may ease the anxiety of seeing your baby's boner for the first time, it won't prepare you for the diapering disasters it can cause. Untamed, urine from a baby's erection can shoot up and stain the ceiling. More explosive than the Fountain of Youth, this forceful expulsion is more akin to a geyser. For obvious reasons, the "tuck technique" is rendered useless in these situations. The best advice for keeping your ceiling urine-free is to minimize your little boy's air time.

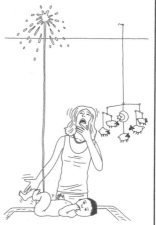

When Nature Calls

Throwing a baseball and baiting a fishing line are time-honored skills passed from father to son. Lesser known but equally important is the tradition of a father teaching his son how to pee in the wilderness.

The typical setting for this proud moment is a park. Your son has just downed a half-bottle of water (at

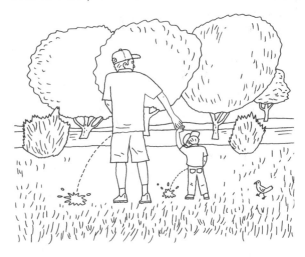

your insistence) on this hot, humid day. After a few bumpy rides on the seesaw, nature has come a-callin'. Your son goes into full pee-pee dance mode, clutching his crotch as you scan the park for a Porta-Potty. No luck.

It's time, you think to yourself. A broad smile comes across your face as you lead your son into the woods. You find a clearing and begin to instruct your son on how to drain the hose without getting his underwear and shoes wet. At first your son is in disbelief that such a transgression would be allowed. He then looks over at you and finds that you, too, are becoming one with nature.

You ignore the chastising stares of moms nearby and enjoy this glorious moment . . . even if your son's shoes happen to be soaking wet.

Spit-Up

Infants do more than eat, poop, sleep, and cry. They also spit up!

Spitting up, like midnight awakenings and dirty diapers, is a universal part of infancy. A dry cleaner's dream, spitting up refers to the spontaneous regurgitation of food and liquid, usually shortly after a meal (and almost always on your freshly pressed shirt).

At first, parents may grow concerned that something is wrong with the breast milk or infant formula. In contrast to this parental anxiety, babies are typically unfazed by this recycling of food. In fact, they are typically ready to eat again and, in general, could care less that they just upchucked the contents of their prior meal (or that they just put another few bucks in your dry cleaner's pocket).

Spitting up is normal in children less than one year of age. It can happen several times a day and usually involves regurgitation of about an ounce of fluid at a time. Larger or more frequent spit-ups should prompt a visit to the doctor.

So why do babies spit up, anyway? Turns out the valve that separates the esophagus from the stomach, known as the lower esophageal sphincter, is weak in young children. This valve's main job is to keep food and liquid in the stomach. After babies have finished gorging on breast milk, their distended stomachs need to decompress. The result is a *wet burp*. If you are lucky, only a droplet or two of milk will make its way up and out. In other situations, it can seem as if the entire stomach has emptied.

Spitting up, especially when large in quantity, is usually followed by a period of ravenous hunger as babies seek to once again refill their now empty tank.

Spitting up peaks at around four months of age and

resolves in 90 percent of kids by the time they hit age one. Not willing to wait a year for Ol' Faithful to stop spewing milk all over the house? Here are some tricks:

1. Hold your baby upright. The seated position can contribute to spitting up because of pressure placed on the stomach caused by bending at the waist.
2. Burp your child, again preferably in the upright position, during and after feedings. This will release air pressure in the stomach.
3. If steps 1 and 2 don't work, try thickening formula with rice cereal to maximize chances it stays in the stomach (the heavier the liquid, the harder it is to reflux).
4. Talk with your child's pediatrician about anti-reflux medications, usually a last resort.
5. If all else fails, at least make sure you have an ample supply of burp cloths.

Vomit

Some would say you haven't experienced parent-hood until you have dealt with a Class III Poonami. Dealing with a bad case of the baby barfs falls into the same parental right-of-passage cat-egory. Poo's effects, even when liquid, are largely mitigated by the use of a diaper, whereas vomit's unconstrained (and unpredictable) nature can result in a greater degree of collateral damage.

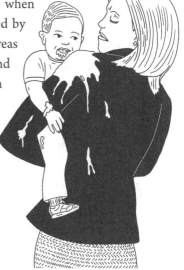

Anyone who has had a bout of food poisoning after eating leftover Chinese food, or too many drinks at a college party, knows what vomiting is. Vomiting involves pressurized expulsion of gastric and intestinal contents via the mouth.

Relatively innocuous, vomiting can often occur after a large meal when a baby has swallowed too much air. As your baby belches to decompress the stomach, most (or all) of the previous feeding can be ejected simultaneously. This is rarely a cause for concern. In this scenario, babies are often hungry and eager to resume feeding almost immediately after throwing up.

The real potential for disaster occurs when your child contracts a viral infection (norovirus and rotavirus, again, are most common). Here the vomiting is severe and repetitive. Parents will feel helpless as they try to curtail the constant barrage of vomit, concerned more about their child's health than the ruined wardrobe. Babies with viral infections do *not* want to eat, and the main concern is dehydration, especially if diarrhea is also present (Double Barrel, page 162).

These infections can have you ducking for cover as projectile vomit flies through the air. If things get really bad, you will find yourself reaching for ski goggles and a rain suit, all the while wondering why there is no diaper equivalent to contain this torrent of vomit (a bib is a sorry excuse).

Survival Tips When Your Child Is Vomiting from a Viral Infection

1. Immediately change your clothes and put on your most dreadful outfit. For dads, this usually involves a hole-ridden college T-shirt. For moms, grab some baggy sweatpants and, well, your own hole-ridden college T-shirt.
2. Layer the changing pad, crib, and play mat with old towels. As towels become contaminated, roll them up and toss them in a bucket of water. Avoid the immediate urge to wash them (there is more vomit on the way!).
3. Try to limit the number of places you put your kid down; if you can limit him to one room, even better.
4. Disrobe your child, except for a diaper. You will have enough to clean in sheets and towels

alone. Plus, removing a contaminated onesie without getting vomit in your baby's hair is nearly impossible.

Now that you have secured the environment, let's turn to your child. Thankfully, most viral infections cause vomiting for less than twenty-four hours. You can try slipping in a teaspoon or two of an oral rehydration solution, like Pedialyte, every five to ten minutes, or have your child suck on a Pedialyte Popsicle. Try to keep your baby upright and resist the urge to give him large quantities of liquids at once (or else get ready for more vomiting).

Pyloric Stenosis

Consistent vomiting after every meal can be a sign of pyloric stenosis, a condition that manifests between four and eight weeks of age. Narrowing of the pyloric muscle at the end of the stomach prevents passage of meal contents into the intestines and leads to projectile vomiting. Milk is vomited forcefully and can literally land on the other side of the room. Surgery is performed to decrease the pressure in this tight muscle, allowing easy passage of milk downstream.

Puke Palette

The Puke Palette is relatively simple when compared to the Poo Palette. Early on, newborns consume only white food (breast milk or formula), so colorful vomit is never due to diet. Later, once they start consuming things like fruit juices and Popsicles, vomit can take on any number of colors.

Green

Bile gives vomit a green color and can be seen with a gastrointestinal infection or an intestinal blockage. If the intestines are blocked, bile will back up into the stomach and be expelled.

Red

This is usually due to blood and may be a cause for concern. An underappreciated and common cause of vomiting blood in newborns is seen when babies swallow blood from small cracks in Mom's nipples. Bleeding is usually small in quantity and resolves once Mom's nipples heal. While there may be benign causes, a good rule of thumb is that if your baby spews blood, you should call your pediatrician.

Black

Blood in the stomach, once mixed with acid, becomes black and looks like coffee grounds. Any black vomit should be considered a sign of bleeding (assuming, of course, your child doesn't drink coffee) and trigger a call to your pediatrician.

Bottom Line: If your child's vomit is the typical yellowish/white, direct your efforts at cleanup and hydration. If the vomit is colorful, especially red or black, without clearly being attributed to a colorful meal your child recently ingested, call your pediatrician.

Double Barrel

If there is a worst-case scenario, this is it. The only thing worse than a barrage of baby barf or a Poonami is a barrage of baby barf *and* a Poonami, *at the same time.* This is Armageddon, an all-hands-on-deck situation that requires cooperation among caregivers and ample supplies. As luck would have it, the same viruses that trigger vomiting also cause massive diarrhea. If you are lucky, you will only have to deal with one issue at a time (usually vomiting first, then diarrhea).

Surviving the Double Barrel involves integrating the survival tips for vomiting (page 157) and the Poonami (page 78). You must contain each bodily emission independently (easier for poo) and quickly clean any environmental contamination.

If there are two caregivers (if you can rope in an unsuspecting younger uncle or aunt, even better), we recommend taking shifts to avoid fatigue and lapses in judgment. Your child's room will end up looking (and smelling) like a war zone and your friends and family may never look at you the same, but there are no style points when it comes to dealing with the Double Barrel. It's about hydration and survival.

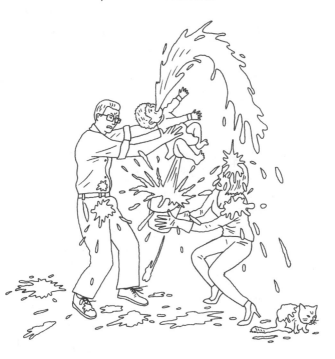

Gas

Ahh . . . glorious gas.

While it often plays second fiddle (or should we say, second horn?) to poo, gas remains an important target of parental attention in the early years. In this section, we give gas, in the forms of farts and burps, some much-needed air time.

As a new parent, it can seem as if gaseous emissions are coming at you from all angles. Your baby will seem like a double-barrel semiautomatic weapon as she fires gas bullets from both ends without regard for propriety. As her backside rests in your hands, you will develop an intimate understanding of the differences between wet farts, machine-gun farts, and the high-pitched toot. You will yearn for the days when you and your spouse would politely stifle belches at the dinner table or scurry to the bathroom to let one rip.

Need further evidence of gas's central role in babyhood? Look no further than the fact that gas has long been blamed as the cause of infant colic, driving parents to eliminate all gas-forming foods from the child's diet. Some nursing mothers go so far as severely restricting their own diets in the hopes that this will soothe their baby's digestive system.

On the other hand, there are times when you welcome, even celebrate, the sound of a gaseous discharge. Being able to efficiently elicit a burp after the 3 AM feeding so you can finally go back to sleep is an important skill needed to survive parenthood. Equally valuable is developing an intuition to quickly sniff out the rancid aroma of a "false alarm" fart from the would-be poopy diaper.

These gassy challenges, and your ability to handle them, will go a long way in determining whether you survive parenthood's early years.

So, read on. It's time to clear the air.

Burps

We spend most of our adult lives trying to avoid gaseous bodily emissions—stifling a belch at a business dinner, taking a well-timed walk to anonymously release a quiet fart, quickly escaping an elevator filled with a coworker's noxious flatulence....

Yet here we are, tired and spent, barely able to keep our eyes open, trying to get Junior to burp so we can

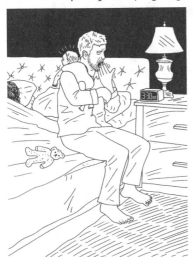

get some much-needed sleep. Many a parent has prayed to hear that little "uuurp" in the middle of the night so that they can safely put their child back to sleep after the midnight feeding.

What begins as a gentle tapping on your baby's back progresses to a firm pat accompanied by verbal "encouragement" and eventual bribery. (*If you burp just this once, I prom- ise I'll read you an extra bedtime story instead of watching the ball game.*)

After fifteen minutes of trying and failing to co- erce the passage of a small amount of air from your baby's stomach, funny things begin to happen. Like a sleep-deprived prisoner, the mind begins to weaken and self-preservation takes over. A desperate parent may gladly convince himself that the creaking of the floorboard or the baby's cough was actually a small burp. Convincing yourself that you really did hear a burp means that your shift in the burping sweatshop is over and sleep can resume.

Why Do We Need to Burp Babies?

Burping involves the forceful passage of air from the stomach in the upward direction, where it is expelled through the mouth. This process releases stomach pressure that has accumulated after eating and drink- ing. Babies younger than four months old are ineffi- cient eaters, meaning they ingest large amounts of air as they suck and swallow. Air is also gulped down in large quantities during fits of crying (which babies do from time to time). This air pressure in the baby's stomach, if not released, can lead to discomfort and the Spit-Up (page 152).

So why can't babies burp on their own, like we do? Turns out they lack the abdominal muscle strength to push out air from their stomachs. This lack of truncal tone means they need a little help to coax air from the GI tract.

Bottom Line: Burping your child after feedings will result in a more comfortable baby and will also decrease the chances of the infamous *wet burp* and its close cousin, the *spit-up*. Spitting up feedings can lead to an unhappy and perpetually hungry baby, not to mention more laundry.

How to Correctly Burp Your Child

Burping is not rocket science. It's also not tackle football. The proper technique involves holding your baby upright and gently patting and/or rubbing his back. Force doesn't matter. Patting harder and faster, turning your child upside down, and bouncing your child on your knee are not going to help. If a reasonable amount of time, say ten to fifteen minutes, has failed to produce a burp, don't worry. One way or another, the air will come out.

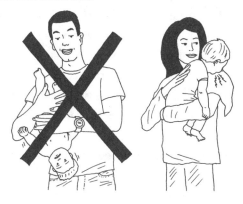

Survival Tip

Stopping in the middle of a feeding may not be popular with your still-hungry baby but can be a good time to elicit a burp.

Farts

The Basics

Gas buildup can be uncomfortable for babies. Its release can be a source of pure joy for the baby and parent alike. In adults, gas formation is almost always related to diet. Not so in newborns. Given their limited diet early in life (either breast milk or formula), most gas formation can be attributed to other things. The leading cause of infant gas is swallowing air during eating (especially in bottle-fed babies) and crying. As discussed elsewhere, some of this air is eliminated by burping; the rest will travel downstream and make a back-door exit.

Formula intolerance and food allergies can lead to a fussy, gassy baby. Improperly digested carbohydrates can make it into the large intestine, where they are fermented by bacteria. This process results in the release of various gases such as hydrogen and carbon dioxide. Use of a different formula, especially one that contains probiotics (healthy bacterial supplements) can improve digestion and spare your child gas attacks.

Knowing the importance of eliminating intestinal air, parents may employ various techniques to help alleviate their baby's gas buildup. Two popular maneuvers are the baby massage and the baby bellows. Massaging of the belly includes both a gentle, circular motion as well as the more extreme downward-pushing technique. Baby bellowing involves gently bringing your child's knees to her chest, followed by extending her legs, and repeating this in a rhythmic fashion. The latter technique is also known as the baby bicycle.

Gas Transmission

One of the common misconceptions regarding infant gas is the role of the mother's diet while breast-feeding. Broccoli, Brussels sprouts, and cabbage? Many moms have been (incorrectly) told to avoid these "gassy" foods for fear that eating them will lead to a gassy and fussy baby. For this to be true, the gas-forming compounds found in these foods would have to somehow end up in breast milk. Turns out, this is physiologically impossible.

The gas pains and flatulence we experience from eating a bushel of broccoli are produced by fermentation occurring in our intestines. Fiber is digested by our intestinal bacteria and eliminated into the atmosphere. Neither gas nor the fibrous substances that cause gas, therefore, pass through breast milk. While a mom's excess flatulence may have drawbacks for her spouse, rest assured that her kid is not suffering.

In some cases, a mother's diet *can* impact her baby's flatulence. Infants may be allergic to foods consumed by Mom, most commonly cow's milk. When milk is ingested, cow's milk proteins are passed along in the breast milk to the baby, where they can cause gastrointestinal distress (Dairy Doo, page 114). In this specific case, eliminating dairy products from the mother's diet will lead to improvement in the baby's symptoms.

Smoke Signal

There is no arguing a fart's deadliest attribute is its aroma. Its sound, after all, is harmless. Some would even call it humorous. Why, then, would a parent covet this horrid stench, which sends passersby running for cover, shirts held tightly over their noses? To understand this seeming paradox we must first define the Smoke Signal.

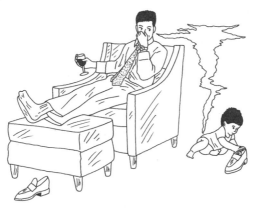

The Smoke Signal, also affectionately known as the Fake-Out Fart, refers to the passage of gas so foul it can trick novice caregivers into thinking a bowel movement has occurred. The typical scenario goes something like this:

After a long, hard day at work (and very little sleep the night before), you plop yourself down in front of the television with a glass of wine. Looking for a thirty-minute respite before the bath and bedtime routine, you can't believe what your nose is telling you. *You've got to be kidding!* The stench emanating from your baby's diaper can only mean one thing: Your little one has dropped a deuce.

Tears begin to form in your eyes as you face the sad reality that your first break all day lasted all of five minutes. You begin to wonder how long a dirty diaper can stay on before either (a) your baby begins freaking out, or (b) he gets a diaper rash (page 82). You glance over at your child and see that he is happily playing and decide to continue with some much-needed "me time."

At the first commercial break, your guilt begins to

mount. You get up, resigned to changing the dirty diaper, when you realize the unpleasant smell has gone. You reach over and pat your child's backside. You may even employ the Dipstick technique (page 98). Sure enough, the vault is empty! *Smoke Signal*, you think to yourself, smiling. You sit back, kick up your feet, and pour yourself another glass of wine.

A well-timed Smoke Signal is one of the true blessings of parenthood. Whether after a long day's work or in the middle of the night, you will soon come to know and yearn for the putrid, poolike aroma of this gas passage, knowing that it has no associated diaper duty.

Fart Fraud, aka Blame the Baby Fart

It is not uncommon for an exhausted parent to let his or her own hygiene take a backseat to a child's health and happiness. Wrinkled dress shirts, tousled hair, and stained clothing don't concern you as much as they once did. You may also grow less concerned about social norms that used to seem important. Sleep-deprived, kid-focused parents, propped up on black coffee, are wont to openly fart without regard for their environment or company.

What do you do the next time someone walks by immediately after you release a smelly fart in the aisle of a grocery store?

Blame your baby. Look at him lovingly, and playfully ask, "Did you just make a poopy?"

Yes, you are throwing your baby under the bus. But, remember, he's the reason you are in this mess to begin with.

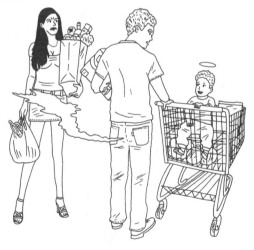

Seven

The Potty Train

Even for the heartiest of poo enthusiasts, there comes a time when you can't bring yourself to change another soggy, smelly diaper. With thousands of diaper changes under your belt, there isn't a color or consistency of poo you haven't seen. Diaper changes on an airplane or at the beach? Been there, done that. Nothing can faze you. That said, it is time to move on. You are ready for a new challenge.

Doosclaimer: If you are still expecting your first baby, or you just had your kid, there are more pressing matters, like figuring out when you can get more than three hours of sleep at a time and how to properly swaddle your baby. Rest assured, there is a light at the end of this tunnel! Read on and file away this information for future reference.

Time to Train the Diaper Champ?

Diapers stink.

Lugging around a bag filled with extra diapers, changing pad, wipes, and diaper cream every time you leave the house is getting old. On your last vacation, half of your suitcase was filled with diaper-changing paraphernalia. You look on with envy while moms of potty-trained kids tote their Chanel clutches as you drag around a monstrous satchel whose shoulder straps have left permanent indentations in your clavicle. That's it, you think. It is time to make the move. Potty training, here we come.

Okay, so wanting a change in handbags is not a valid reason to usher in the potty-training era. Turns out your child's age may not be the best indicator, either. Research has shown that there is a wide range of what constitutes an appropriate age to teach Junior to tinkle in the toilet. Factors such as gender, development, birth order, and culture all factor into determining when your little one will jump on the throne.

Here are some diaper-bursting facts:

- The Greatest Generation: 90 percent of American toddlers growing up in the early 1900s were potty trained by age two (today, it's less than 10 percent).
- Potty training begins at age six months in certain developing Asian and African countries, with most children fully potty trained by age one.
- Freudian gift? Diaper companies have neurologist Sigmund Freud to thank for their billion-dollar business. His proclamation in the early 1900s that early and forceful potty training can lead to long-term psychological problems is the reason most children are in diapers longer.

The Disappearing Act

During the first couple of years of your child's life, he will seemingly poop anywhere, anytime, without breaking stride. As he gets older, however, the style and substance of poo begins to evolve. While some poo will remain small, others are monster poos so large you'll wish they were yours (Poo Envy, page 138). Similarly, your child's emissions will become so pungent that you will be left wondering how someone so small can create something so foul.

One of the most intriguing times during a baby's pooping evolution begins when he starts to quietly slip away to poop in a corner. Seemingly overnight, your child goes from dropping the deuce in the middle of a dinner party to sneaking away for a private poopy break.

This change in poo practice is often the first sign that your child may be ready for potty training. (Knowing when you have to go to the bathroom is half the battle.) At a certain age, children begin to realize that moving your bowels is a private activity.

While some parents stick to positive reinforcement, aka bribery, by giving a child one M&M's candy for peeing in the toilet and two M&M's for pooping, others utilize more unorthodox potty-training tactics. These include:

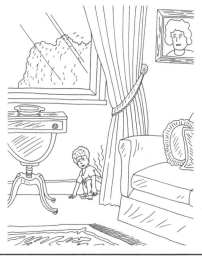

- **The "Free Method"**: Some bold parents employ commando training, allowing their tot to stroll around unhindered from the waist down ("Honey, tell me he didn't just drop one on the Persian?!").

- **The "Denim Style"**: This practice involves dressing a child in cheap denim jeans without a diaper in order to make peeing and pooping anywhere but the toilet so uncomfortable that children will only want to relieve themselves on the potty. Denim Style practitioners will do a lot more laundry, and clean a lot more pee (and poop) off the floor, but this technique unquestionably accelerates a child's transition to using the toilet.

- **"Elimination Communication"**: Elimination communication (EC) is when a caregiver attempts to use timing and signals to address an infant's need to pee or poop. Caregivers try to recognize and respond to a baby's need to eliminate waste. Some practitioners of EC, particularly in the developing world, begin soon after birth, although it can be started at any age.

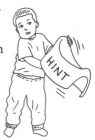

Bottom Line: Private poo is a good thing! It means your life free of diapers (at least until you have another kid) is potentially just around the corner. Next time your child scurries away with that about-to-poop look on his face, try to redirect him to the bathroom.

Poop Trail

It would be nice if the path to becoming potty trained was linear (it's not). At first, you are happy if your child lets you know when he has to use the bathroom (this is immediately followed by a mad dash to the toilet).

Later on, your child may walk himself to the loo and plop down on the throne and start taking care of business. This is liberating because (*finally*) you don't have to drop everything the moment Junior gives the go signal.

But don't lag too far behind. While your child may now know when he has to go to the bathroom, he may not always know when he is *done* going to the bathroom. It is not uncommon to discover a Poop Trail from your bathroom if your child has prematurely left the throne, usually after being summoned by a playmate or hearing the return of his favorite TV character.

If the job is not yet done, buttock inspection will

reveal poop particles in mid-exit—the so-called Hanging Chads or Klingons. When you are young, it is apparently more important to get back to life than to have a clean butt.

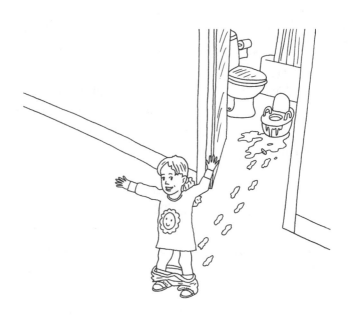

Survival Tip

Encourage your child to go to the bathroom on his own but stay close by. This way, if he decides to make a premature exit, you are there to intervene. Teach him the importance of wiping. His current playmates may not care if he is covered in poop, but there's a good chance his future friends will.

Too Big for Your Britches?

Even among friends, there is healthy (?) competition between parents. *My child rolled over at three months! Mine slept through the night at four months. . . .*

One of the biggest milestones to be openly celebrated is when your child becomes potty trained. This accomplishment is broadcasted far and wide for all to know. Parents may dress their child in tight-fitting pants to show off the absence of a diaper butt. Moms will conspicuously tote their petite clutch during a visit to a friend's house to highlight her lack of a diaper bag.

Parents of the newly potty trained: Remain humble in your newfound freedom from diapers and wipes.

The early days of a potty-trained child can be fraught with accidents. And if you just strolled in, head held high, flaunting your new life free from poop, don't ex-

pect any sympathy when your child pees through her
white tights in the middle of dinner.

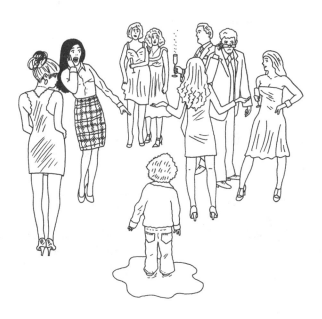

Bottom Line: Accidents happen. When the com-
mitment is made to go without diapers, be steadfast
but not cocky. It is likely that your kid will have an

accident when and where you least expect it. Puddles on your friend's floor, in a hotel lobby, or in the middle of a crowded restaurant are some of the classic post–potty-training mishaps. For your child's sake, remain positive when accidents occur and rest assured that this phase, too, will quickly pass.

Survival Tip

No matter how confident you are that your child has successfully conquered potty training, hold on to that diaper bag for a little while longer. Bring extra underwear and clothing for the first few months of diaper-free living, even if you are determined to show off your child's latest achievement (and your new purse).

Eight

Bottoms Up!

Whether you have successfully potty trained your child or are still having trouble distinguishing the front from the back of a diaper, you know that having a child means putting up with a lot of crap. Your baby's bodily waste can take over your life, but only if you let it. We hope this book makes raising your baby a tad easier and a lot more enjoyable.

Poo teaches us many important parenting lessons. It reminds us to be humble and flexible. Wayward poop can ruin an elegant dress or stylish sport coat, while an unexpected baby blowout can disrupt the most tightly planned travel itinerary.

Most important, baby poo will teach you to go with the flow and to laugh amid the sleep deprivation and stress involved in raising a child. What else can you do when confronted with a Class III Poonami that has left poo in your baby's hair? How about that monstrous expulsion of baby gas in the middle of your child's preschool interview?

Surviving this barrage of bodily waste may sometimes mean finishing that glass of wine before changing your baby's dirty diaper. He'll live, and you'll live happier. Hit square in the eyeball by your son's Fountain of Youth? Laugh it off. It happens to the best of us. After all, urine is sterile and you now have great material for your toast at your son's wedding.

One day (a long, long time from now) you might actually look back at all this and miss it.

Then again, maybe you won't.

Either way, enjoy the ride.

Josh Richman was born and raised in Philadelphia, Pennsylvania, to a family with a rich history in the plumbing industry. His great-grandfather, grandparents, and two uncles were in the plumbing supply business and Josh fondly remembers the days he spent in 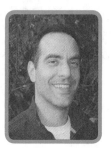 high school working at the family plumbing supply store. Josh attended Brown University, where he became friends with his then classmate and now writing partner, Anish Sheth. After a stint working in Washington, DC, Josh moved to the San Francisco Bay Area, where he now lives with his wife and two kids.

Anish Sheth holds undergrad-
uate and medical degrees from
Brown University and is currently
a gastroenterologist in Princeton,
New Jersey. His obsession with
poo can be traced back to childhood conversations held at the
family dinner table regarding bow-

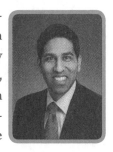

el movements. He lives in Princeton with his wife and
two children, and is happy to report that his diaper-
changing days are behind him.

The Poo Palette

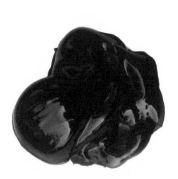

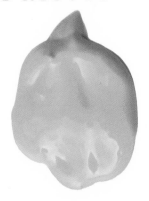

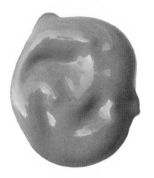

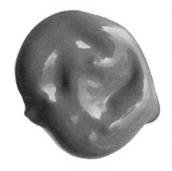